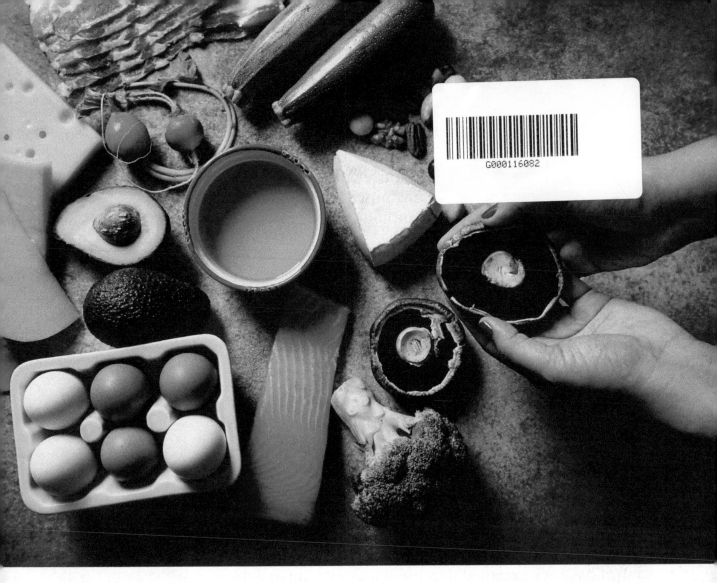

KETO DIET COOKBOOK FOR WOMEN AFTER 50

THE MOST COMPLETE KETOGENIC DIET MANUAL
REBOOT YOUR METABOLISM AND BOOST YOUR ENERGY WITH 200
AFFORDABLE AND EASY RECIPES AND A 21-DAY MEAL PLAN

Nigella Jennifer Willett

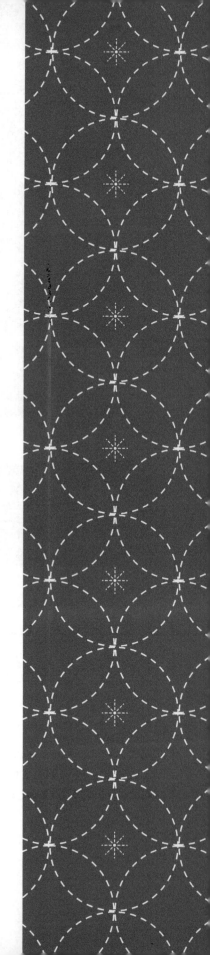

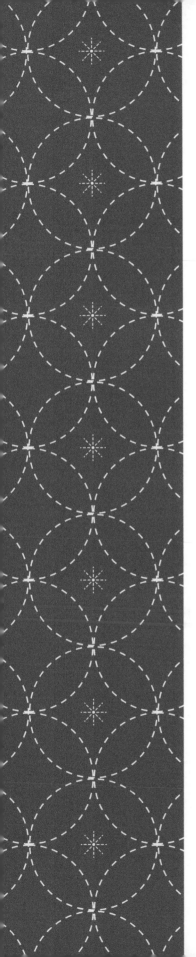

TABLE OF CONTENTS

CHAPTER 3
HOW TO CUSTOMIZE YOUR KETO DIET

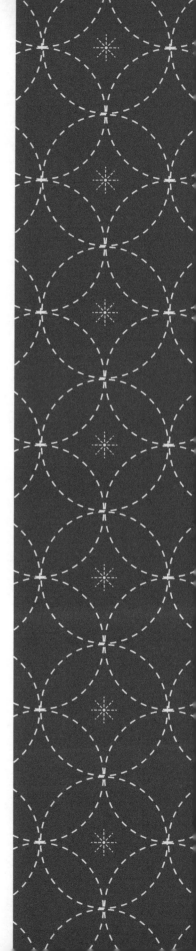

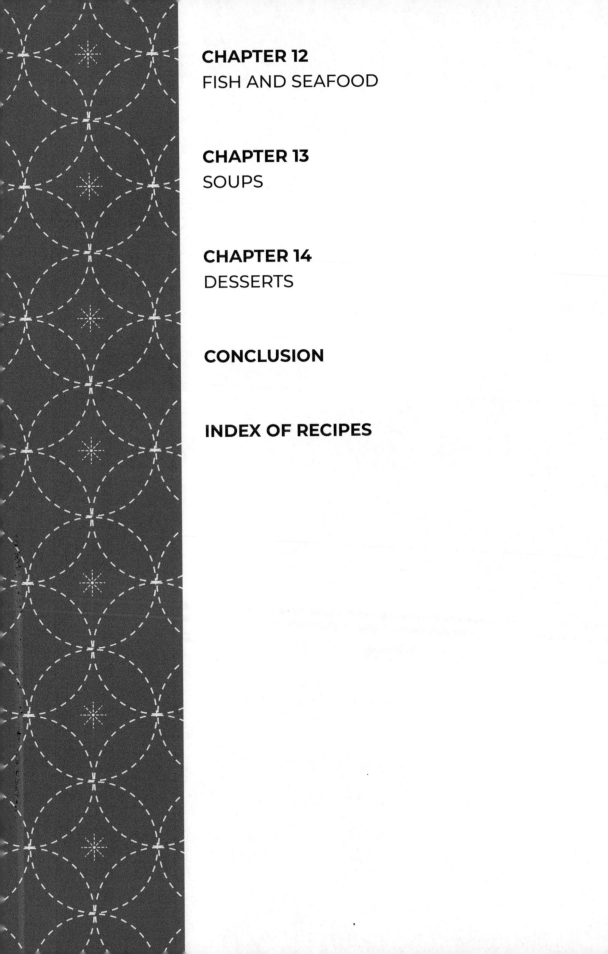

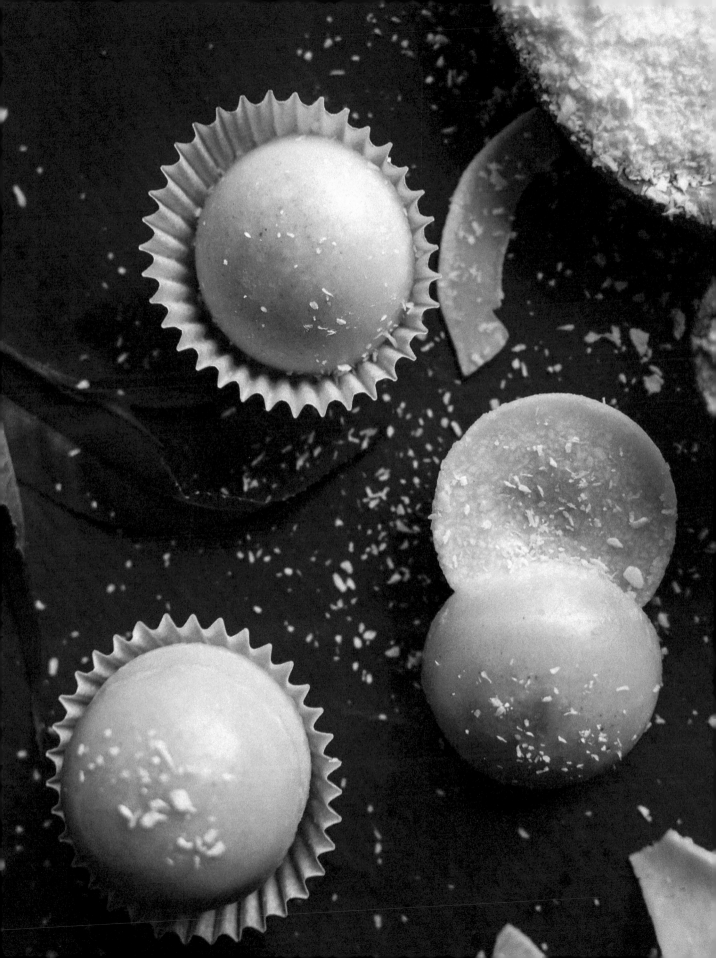

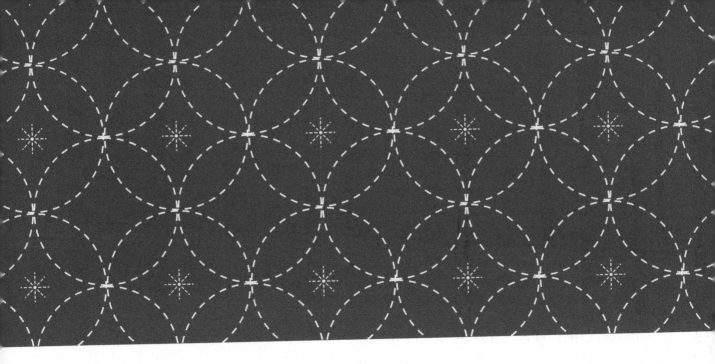

INTRODUCTION

Each of us is unique, which is why the most effective diet plan for any woman is one that is tailor-made to meet her personal needs. If you are to maximize your health and well-being you have to know how best to do this at your particular stage in life and in your particular situation.

The good news is that working out a health-care plan that matches the complexity of your life is not impossible. With a little research, guides to follow and a mindset geared towards success, you'll be on your way to a healthier you in no time.

As we age, it becomes more imperative that we obtain as much information as possible in order to embrace a lifestyle that encourages good health and helps create a sense of well-being. Women over 50 have shown a great interest in gaining as much information as possible in order to sustain their current health and to make sensible choices about their lifestyles and behaviors. This natural curiosity helps us to acquire new eating habits and modify our exercise routines in order to ensure a more satisfying and longer life. We turn our attention to medical research on nutrition and nutritional needs in order to learn as much as possible about our own health and how to care for our bodies. The results are finally provided, it often seems as though the medical community is playing a game of Russian roulette and the findings seem to change like the seasons.

It can be frustrating when things you thought were right are turned inside-out as new findings come to light. One moment you are told to eat more carbohydrates, and the next you're told that carbohydrates are the cause of your excess weight. Knowledge from medical research usually builds up only slowly, and sometimes it changes completely as more information becomes available.

What you'll find here is the most up-to-date information on how to create and maintain a healthy lifestyle. The keto diet has been around for a very long time and has been proved to be one of the most comprehensive eating plans to not only help you lose unwanted pounds but to help you create a life-long way of eating that will ensure the best of health for years to come.

THE SCIENCE BEHIND THE DIET

One of the toughest things to do when starting any diet is choosing which diet to start. There are literally hundreds of diets to choose from at any given time. A few examples are the dash diet, which was designed to help people lower their high blood pressure. The Mediterranean Diet was developed to reflect food patterns typical of Crete, Greece and southern Italy; the Flexitarian Diet was developed to help people reap the benefits of a vegetarian diet while still enjoying animal products in moderation; and of course, America's most famous, Weight Watchers diet. Each of these diets makes promises of all kinds including effortless weight loss without sacrifice and without hunger. They offer quick results with minimal effort. They share their gimmicks, tricks, and hooks to get you excited enough to begin, but fall short of explaining the science behind their promises. Usually, because there is no science. Just fad after fad that someone has thought up to make money. You know how their story ends. You start, you fall, you fail. And you end up right back where you started, very often, having added a couple of extra pounds to top it all off.

The keto diet is much more than a fad diet; it will actually teach you a new way of eating that is not just for the time being, but forever. The science is flawless, the results have proven time and time again. It is a completely new way of eating that is not just for the moment—but is sustainable for a lifetime. You will be training your body to treat food in a whole new way.

The keto diet was originally developed by researchers and doctors for children with epilepsy. Studies proved that this special high-fat, very low-carb and protein plan helped to control, if not eliminate, seizures in children and adults with this debilitating disease. Over the course of the studies, it was noted that the patient's weights were affected in a positive way.

Let's take a moment and reflect on what we are actually talking about here. The word "diet" has such a negative connotation in today's world. It brings to mind images of celery sticks and carrots, starvation, and a never-ending struggle with will power. It implies that someone has issues with eating habits, most specifically, overeating. But that's not what the word should mean to us. If you check a dictionary, you'll find that the word diet is simply a reference to the type of foods that a person, community, or animal habitually eats.

Let's begin by embracing the idea that the keto diet is not really a "diet" at all, but merely a habitual way of eating to create a healthy body. We aren't going to "restrict" our foods, we may eliminate some, and we may control portions on others, but we will not think of our new-way-of-eating as depriving ourselves—but instead, that we are creating a pathway to a more healthy and happy body, and consider this new-way-of-eating as the right path to lead us towards that goal.

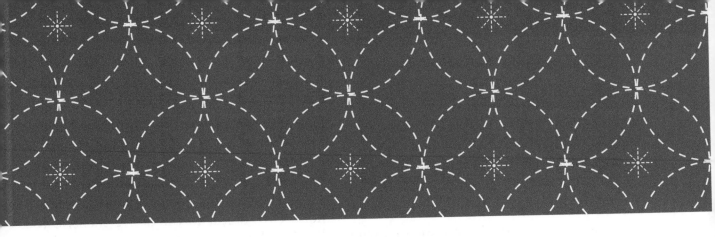

CHAPTER 1
WHAT IS THE KETOGENIC DIET, THE BENEFITS OVER 50

WHAT IS KETOSIS?

The ketogenic diet comprises high fat, enough protein, and a minimal carbohydrate diet. Keto makes it necessary for the body to burn fats as compared to carbohydrates. The body will go into a state known as ketosis. Ketosis is a metabolic state. It mainly occurs when the body does not have sufficient access to glucose. Glucose is the primary source of energy for the organization.

When the body lacks glucose, acid is developed and is known as ketones. The question now is, why the ketogenic diet? How is keto beneficial to our health? Keto diet transforms fat into ketones in the liver, charged with the responsibility of supplying energy for the brain. Your body will also become incredibly efficient at burning fat for energy. This kind of diet can sometimes lead to reduced blood sugar and reduced level of insulin. While under the ketogenic diet, you will also have a better and deeper sleep. You will have more energy the whole day and will still feel full, not like many low carb diets.

"Metabolism" is a common word in the modern world, and the chances are high that it is not your first time hearing this word since your childhood. The issues are, do you really understand what it means? It defines chemical reactions in the body of a living organism, ensuring normal functioning hence normal life. Unquestionably, human beings have a simple metabolism despite the complications of their bodies. Human bodies are ever at work no matter the situation they are in, be it; while sleeping, the cells are ever in the process of reforming. The energy they use in building and reforming is extracted from the body itself.

The outcome of carbohydrate digestion— Glucose, is the building power of metabolism. Many books out there emphasize on various Nutrition guidelines recommending how carbohydrates as the father of energy.

KETOSIS AND THE KETOGENIC DIET

As described above, what then is ketosis? It is a metabolic state. A state where the body is in short of enough glucose; therefore, less energy, burns stored fat instead; this leads to the accumulation of acids called ketones within the body.

Ketosis thrives in conditions such as when the body does not have sufficient access to glucose. It usually takes only two days for your body to go into ketosis, so make sure to follow your ketogenic diet properly, and you will reach the health benefits that come with keto a lot quicker.

THE DIFFERENT TYPES OF KETOGENIC DIETS

Firstly, we need to understand different distinctions in the keto diet. The majority believe that there is only one ketogenic diet. In reality, there are four types of ketogenic diets. Despite their similarity, they possess some variances in the macronutrient content.

The first to begin with is the standard ketogenic diet. It is all about fat intake; it has a macronutrient ratio of 75% fat, equivalent to about 150 grams of fat a day, which will result in the switch of your metabolism to now burn fat as fuel. You will also need about five to 10% of carbs in a single day, translating to about only 50 grams of carbs, and you will finally need 15-20% of protein, which also translates to around 90 grams in a single day or 30 grams per meal, which is equivalent to four ounces of meat.

The second type is a targeted Keto diet. Targeted Keto diet is mostly popular amongst athletes. For this type of food, you will have an additional 20-30 grams of carbs in a single day. Its macronutrient breakdown is 65 to 70% fat, 10-15% carbs, and 20% of protein. The carb intake of this diet is about 70 to 80 grams in a single day. About 20 to 30 grams of carbs before going for a workout and after going for conditioning to ensure better recovery as well as a higher intensity workout. However, you should not worry about the fact that you will be kicked out of keto. Give credit to the active lifestyle you live in. The extra carbs you consume will be broken down during the workout.

The third type is the cyclical keto diet. Cyclical keto diet calls for an individual having five days of the traditional keto diet and two non-keto days in a very week. The macronutrient ratio on its keto days is 75% fat, 5-10% carbs, and 15 to 20% protein. On non-keto days, the macronutrient ratio is 25% that 50% carbs, and 25% of protein. You can use special occasions like graduation parties, birthdays, or other significant events to adopt the non-keto days.

THE CHARACTERISTICS OF THE KETOGENIC DIET

There are ten main features of the ketogenic diet. It helps in maintaining and improving lean body mass and performance. Being on a ketogenic diet does not make it necessary for calorie counting. Calorie counting is not relevant for the accomplishment of weight loss; all you need to pay attention to is the number of carbs you consume.

When our body is weak with less entry due to a shortage of glucose, the body will burn a lot of fats hence store lots of fats. This results in the accumulation of acids called ketones within the organization. Ketosis is the metabolic state when this happens. The ketogenic diet is majorly comprised of whole, healthy fruits as well as providing adequate macronutrients to preserve lean body mass and function. The macronutrient levels vary as there are four types of ketogenic diets. No matter which ketogenic diet you pick, make sure to follow the macronutrient chart.

The ketogenic diet has sufficient intercellular minerals and electrolytes to maintain quality, muscle, nerve, and circulatory functions. Unlike most diets, the ketogenic diet does not exactly follow the usual dietary guidelines. If you choose a ketogenic diet, and you have chronic conditions, for example, diabetes or hypertension, make sure to have ongoing medical supervision for medication management. The ketogenic diet has a lot of essential characteristics to help you decide whether this diet is right for you or not.

The ketogenic diet is not a modern invention. It has existed since. From past experiences, it has been realized that if a person with epilepsy fasts, or rather stops eating, their seizures usually stop. The very first scientific study on fasting for the treatment of epilepsy was done in France in 1910. According to the survey, it was realized that that seizures stopped during the period of absolute fasting. In later evaluations, cessation of seizures was observed, as well as an improvement in mental activity during starvation. However, a person can't last indefinitely.

As of 1924, Dr. Peterman, at the Mayo Clinic, regularly adopted the diet, and the treatment was adopted widely around the 1930s. After the Second World War, Dr. Livingston examined around 1000 patients with the keto diet and was amazed by the marvelous seizure control. With time, innovative and more actual anti-seizure medications were developed, declining interest in the ketogenic diet.

Approaching the end of the 1980s, attention towards the diet was invigorated by Dr. John Freeman at Johns Hopkins, who conducted a study in 1992 and gave out reports indicating how the food produced complete seizure control in 30% of children with uncontrolled seizures. Charlie Abrahams was one of the children who were among the participants who were treated successfully by the Johns Hopkins team. In appreciation, his parents established the Charlie Foundation. This foundation has provided publicity to the diet in many ways, such as availing free videotape on the subject. While you are free from work, ensure you enjoy some wholesome carb-rich foods as an alternative to processed foods. Consider some whole grains, fruits, and starchy vegetables.

The final type of ketogenic diet is the high protein ketogenic diet. The menu has a macronutrient ratio of 60-65% fat, which will be about 130 grams of fat, 5-10% of carbs, and 30% of protein, which is about 120 grams of protein in one day. From this, you can notice how your carb intake is still restricted.

Try out the keto diet today, and you will find the menu more comfortable than the standard ketogenic diet. This is possible due to your ability to eat more protein and less fat. Another side of this diet that it may not result in ketosis since protein can be turned into glucose for fuel, although there is still a possibility for weight loss. In case you are taking a lot of protein, make sure to track the amount of value intake as you do not want to put yourself out of ketosis, and you do not want to get other adverse effects, as in the keto flu. Because there are four types of ketogenic diets, ensure you note down the advantages and disadvantages of each food for the more natural selection of what suits you.

WHY WE GO, KETO

Why should someone choose keto instead of another type of diet? Does a ketogenic diet have that many benefits? The ketogenic diet has some positive effects. It can mend extreme health conditions such as cardiovascular disease, diabetes, and metabolic syndrome, or even reduce the possibility of contracting cancer. Another benefit of Keto is its ability to improve levels of HDL cholesterol, commonly referred to as good cholesterol, better as compared to other diets with carbohydrates.

It also aids in primary treatment and control of severe epilepsy in children to help reduce their seizures. Some studies have also suggested that the diet could also benefit adults with epilepsy. Another reason people choose the ketogenic diet is; because the ketogenic diet can help you lose much more weight than a low-fat diet while still being able to fill full.

The ketogenic diet also helps to reduce anxiety and depression. Keto also increases and provides sustain energy, reduces inflammation, and balances hormones. This approach has a lot of health benefits. Do more research to ensure that your type of ketogenic diet well suits you.

THE BENEFITS OF KETOSIS

Do you know the health benefits of the ketogenic diet? Others are cognitive; hence, better focus; you will maintain healthy heart functions and general healthy cognitive function. The physical will also be there from the ketogenic diet. Its physical benefits are so significant as they help overcome usual life challenges. Assuming you are suffering from acne, you will notice a reduction in acne as well as experience weight loss. Much weight will be lost in the first week because

your car and water quantity reduce.

How about the psychological benefits of the ketogenic diet? Ketones are considered as fuel, and due to their fuel nature, they improve brain function. You will also have a better and deeper sleep. It will also improve your heart health. The ketogenic diet reduces blood sugar and insulin levels, which is why it is a proper diet for people with diabetes. The ketogenic diet can also potentially reduce the seizures in children and is therapeutic for several brain disorders.

The ketogenic diet is also effective against metabolic syndrome. You will also have an increase in HDL cholesterol, also known as the good cholesterol; your appetite would also reduce. On the ketogenic diet, people swear by the fact that they still feel full, unlike the lowest carbohydrate diets. The ketogenic diet may even lower blood pressure. As you can see, the ketogenic diet has a lot of different health benefits and can also help you reach your health and physical goals.

Some symptoms may be excessive thirst, nausea and vomiting, abdominal pain, fatigue, confusion, and shortness of breath. More specific signs are high ketone levels in your urine and high blood sugar level. Make sure to contact a doctor as soon as possible if you're unable to tolerate food or liquid, you're vomiting, and if the level of ketones in your urine is high. You should also call a doctor if your blood sugar level is higher than usual. Though ketoacidosis is not common among people with diabetes, it still occurs. When you notice these warnings, consult your doctor for further directions.

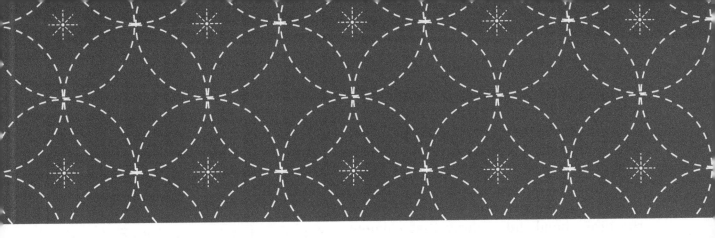

CHAPTER 2
FOCUS ON PEOPLE OVER 50

WHY IS IT IMPORTANT FOR PEOPLE OVER 50?

As you grow in age, the body's natural fat-burning ability reduces. When that happens, your body stops receiving a healthy dose of nutrients properly, which is why you will develop diseases and ailments. With the keto diet, you are pushing the body into ketosis and bypassing the need to worry about your body's ability to burn fat. Once in ketosis, your body will now burn fat forcefully for survival.

Once more, your system will now start to regain strength. An even better aspect that follows is your insulin level because it drops. If you are someone diagnosed with diseases such as type 2 diabetes and others, the drop in insulin might even reverse the effects and eliminate the diseases from your body altogether.

There are studies underway, and most of them suggest that the keto diet is far more beneficial to those above 50 than it is for those under this age bracket. A quick search on Google and you are immediately overwhelmed with over 93 million results, most of which explain the benefits of the keto diet for people above 50. That is a staggering number for a diet plan that has only been around a few years.

It is also important to highlight that as we get older, we start losing more than just the ability to burn fat. During this phase of our life, once we hit around 50 years of age, we come across various obstacles, some chronic in nature, which transpire only because our body is no longer able to function at rates like it did when we were young. Ketogenic diets help us regain that edge and feel energized from within.

There are hundreds of thousands of stories, all pointing out how this revolutionary diet is especially helpful for older adults and the elderly. It is, therefore, a no-brainer for people above 50 who have spent ages trying to search for a healthy lifestyle choice of diet. With such a high success rate, there is no harm in trying, right?

Before the keto phenomenon, there was the Atkins diet. The Atkins diet was also a low carb diet, just like its keto counterpart. This form of diet also became a huge hit with the masses. However, unlike keto, the Atkins diet provided weight loss while putting a person through constant hunger. Keto, on the other hand, takes away that element, and it does that using ketosis.

Constant exposure to ketosis reduces appetite, hence taking away the biggest hurdle in most diets. The Atkins diet failed to address that front, which is why it was more of a hit and miss. However, credit where it is due, the Atkins diet did garner quite a bit of fame. However, since the inception of keto, things have changed dramatically.

A study was conducted where 34 overweight adults were monitored and observed for 12 months. All of them were put on keto diets. The end result showed that participants had lower HgbA1c (hemoglobin A1c) levels, experienced significant weight loss, and were more likely to completely discontinue their medications for diabetes.

All in all, the keto diet is shaping up to be quite a promising candidate for older adults. Not only will this diet allow us to lead a healthier lifestyle, but it will also curb our ailments and ensure high energy around the clock. That is quite the resume for a diet and one that now seems too attractive to pass up. This is the point where I made up my mind and decided to give the keto diet a go, and I recommend the same to you.

Whether you are a man or a woman, if you have put on weight, or you are suffering from ailments like type 2 diabetes, consider this as your ticket to a care-free world where you will lead a healthy life and rise out of the

ailments eventually.

Keto has been producing results that have attracted the top minds and researchers for a fairly long time. Considering the unique nature of this lifestyle of eating, the results have been rather encouraging.

"Great! How do I start?"

Not so fast. While the keto diet is simple, there are a few things I should point out which you should know. Some of these might even change your mind about the entire keto diet plan, but if you are determined for a healthy lifestyle and a fit body, I assure you these should not be of much trouble.

PREPARING YOURSELF FOR KETO

When entering the world of keto, quite a few of us just pick up a recipe on the internet and start cooking things accordingly. While that is good, we do tend to search for any specifics which we should know of, such as what would happen if I replace nuts with something else? Is oatmeal a part of the keto diet? What are keto-approved food items? Are there any risks involved?

Here is some more information regarding such questions:

- Keto is an extremely strict food diet where you can only eat things that can be classified as keto worthy. Anything that falls out of this category is a straight "no!"

- Keto is a completely new lifestyle. That means your body will undergo some changes. While most of these will be good, some may pose problems such as the keto flu. Most of the people I know, including myself, faced this "flu" with similar symptoms to influenza. It was only after some research that I realized this was natural. The keto flu isn't exactly alarming, but it is best to be mentally prepared for it.

- You will need to work on your cooking skills as keto strictly pushes processed, high carb foods out of the diet.

- If you aren't really into the idea of protein and fat intake, you may wish to reconsider as these are the two primary areas keto focuses on.

- Apart from this, there are some mistakes people tend to make when they begin their journey. Some of the most common mistakes are:

- Not knowing the keto food properly: Just because something looks like a keto-friendly item doesn't mean it is keto-approved. Always refer to some food guide to check if the item you are interested in is a part of the "good food" in keto.

- Keeping the same level of fat intake throughout: This often leads to results that show in the start and then disappear. You need to constantly adjust your diet and monitor your protein and fat intake.

- Consuming bullet-proof coffee when you really shouldn't: This coffee involves a mixture of coconut oil and butter within the coffee. While it is a perfect way to keep hunger at bay, it does push the level of bad cholesterol upwards. If you are someone who has been advised to stick to lower cholesterol levels and avoid consuming similar food items, keep this one off the limits.

- Thinking the keto flu is the only issue to face: There are other difficulties that will emerge within the first 10 weeks of your keto journey. This will include lethargic limbs, which will make walking difficult at first. Owing to the change in fiber intake, you may either face diarrhea or constipation as well.

- Pushing bodies with vigorous exercises: You have just started keto, give your body a bit of time to adjust. Keep things slow and steady.

- Not replenishing on electrolytes: Since we mentioned diarrhea and exercise, your body will run low on electrolytes faster than usual. This is something that you may want to keep in check. Think of sodium and potassium!

These are some of the most common mistakes people have made, and surprisingly, even I was no exception. If only I had someone to properly guide me back then.

Now then, you know the "what" and the "how" of keto, but you are yet to figure out whether this diet is meant for women or men. As a part of the first step, I will now provide you more details regarding both the aspects and give you a breakdown of facts to show just how beneficial this diet is for both.

ALLOWED PRODUCT LIST

If you've decided to go on Keto after 50, be sure you won't regret your choice! So when you start something new, the first and the main thing you need to do is consult the Keto dietary features. But most importantly, you must look at the list of allowed products to remember this list and adhere strictly to it.

Don't worry! The low-carb eating plan isn't overly limited. Check out what products you can and must buy in the supermarket and start a new phase in your life.

MEAT AND POULTRY

Chicken, beef, pork, lamb, turkey, veal include no-carb, but high protein and fat intake. That is the primary reason why meat and poultry products are known as staples for the Ketogenic diet. Besides this, bacon and organ meats are also allowed for consumption.

SEAFOOD

When it comes to seafood, you also have an excellent list. You can buy and cook a lot of delicious dishes from:

- Lobster
- Shrimp
- Octopus
- Salmon
- Tuna
- Oysters
- Mussels
- Squid
- Scallops

The most useful Keto seafood is the crab and shrimp. They don't contain carbohydrates at all.

VEGETABLES

Only low-carb and non-starchy veggies can be eaten by the people who go on the Keto diet. This means that you can add the following vegetables:

- Avocados
- Tomatoes
- Cucumbers
- Zucchini
- Radishes
- Mushrooms
- Eggplant
- Celery
- Bell peppers
- Herbs
- Asparagus
- Kohlrabi
- Mustard
- Spinach
- Lettuce
- Kale
- Brussel sprouts

DAIRY PRODUCTS

You should be careful with dairy. Not all dairy food can be useful for you if you want to stick to the Keto diet. Here are the products you can buy and cook:

- Eggs
- Butter and ghee
- Heavy cream and whipping cream
- Sour cream
- Unflavored Greek yogurt
- Cottage cheese
- Hard, semi-hard, soft, and cream cheeses

BERRIES

Unfortunately, most fruits have high levels of carbs and can't be included in the Keto diet. However, you can consume:

- Blackberries
- Raspberries
- Strawberries
- Blueberries

NUTS AND SEEDS

A lot of experts recommend paying attention to nuts and seeds that are high-fat and low-carb. You can add such nuts and seeds to your dishes as:

- Almond
- Pecans
- Walnuts
- Hazelnuts
- Brazil nuts
- Pumpkin seeds
- Sesame seeds
- Chia seeds
- Flaxseed

COCONUT AND OLIVE OILS

To cook tasty fatty dishes, you need oil. Coconut and olive oils have unique properties that make them suitable for a Keto diet. These oils are rich in fat and boost ketone production. Moreover, they can be used for salad dressing and adding to cooked dishes.

LOW-CARB DRINKS

The Keto diet means that you should drink only unsweetened coffee and tea because they don't include carbs and fasten metabolism. Besides, you can drink dark chocolate and cocoa. Such drinks have low levels of carbohydrates, and that's why they're permitted.

PROHIBITED PRODUCT LIST

When it comes to the lists of foods you should avoid on the low-carb, high-fat diet, be attentive and check it carefully. Well, you can't eat:

- Grains (like oatmeal, pasta, bulgur, corn, wheat, buckwheat, rice, etc.)

- Low-fat dairy (fat-free yogurt, skim milk, skim Mozzarella, etc.)

- Most fruits (melon, watermelon, apples, peaches, bananas, grapes, oranges, plums, grapefruits, mangos, cherries, pineapples, pears, etc.)

- Starchy veggies (potatoes, beets, turnips, parsnips, etc.)

- Grain foods (pasta, popcorn, muesli, cereal, bagels, bread, etc.)

- Some oils (soybean oil, grapeseed oil, sunflower oil, peanut oil, canola oil)

- Typical snack foods (crackers, potato chips, etc.)

- Trans fats (margarine.)

- Sweets (candies, buns, pastries, cakes, chocolate, puddings, cookies.)

- Sweeteners and added sugars (corn syrup, cane sugar, honey, agave nectar, etc.)

- Sweetened drinks (sweetened coffee and tea, juice, soda, smoothies.)

- Alcohol (sweet wines, cider, beer, etc.)

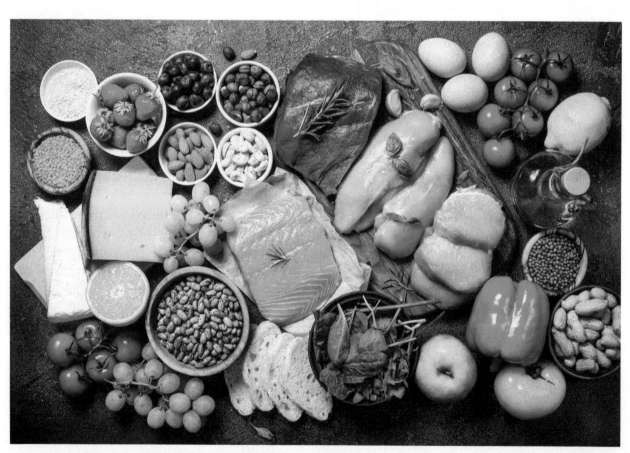

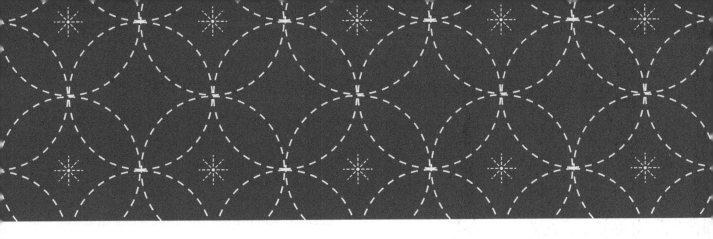

CHAPTER 3
HOW TO CUSTOMIZE YOUR KETO DIET

There are many options when it comes to structuring your daily meals. The bottom line is that there is no one-size-fits-all approach for this, and it really comes down to your schedule, eating habits, and ultimately what allows you to feel most satisfied while maintaining a balanced Keto macro intake.

Once you're past the first week and getting the hang of consuming fewer carbohydrates, adequate-protein, and more healthy fats, you will most likely start to feel more satiated and notice that you can go for more extended periods without eating or snacking while you can still maintaining high energy, mood, and focus levels.

Make it a lifestyle. Figure out the meal timing that fits your schedule, keep you feeling satisfied throughout the day, and allows you to enjoy your meals without triggering more stressors.

The switch from a sugar burner to a fat burner can take some time. Most of us have been running on carbohydrates and sugar our entire lives, and our bodies have no idea what it feels like to be in "fat-burning mode" indeed.

There are a few different phases that our bodies go through during the adjustment period to becoming Keto-adapted. Making sure you take the appropriate steps during each of these phases is crucial for long-term success. During this challenge, you will transition through phase 1 and into phase 2. Phase 3 will come with time.

PHASE 1: GETTING INTO KETOSIS
Achieving ketosis may take about 2-3 days. But the transition can be challenging if you are not taking advantage of the proper tools. Be sure always to follow the rules and guidelines.

1. CUT THE CARBS
The first step toward producing ketones is to decrease the consumption of carbs. Aim for 30 grams or less of total carbs per day and adjust accordingly.

2. CONSUMED ENOUGH HEALTHY FATS

Throw your fear of fat foods out the window and pump your body with the fuel it needs for energy—fat! This will make the transition phase more effective in burning fat

3. MODERATE PROTEIN

Consuming too much protein, especially on its own, may spike insulin levels and make it harder to get into ketosis. Pair proteins with fats and be mindful of your intake.

4. REPLENISH ELECTROLYTES AND WATER

When your intakes of carbs are decreased, your body will start flushing out more water and takes sodium and other electrolytes with it. This can lead to symptoms of "Keto flu," which is in more detail here.

5. AVOID A SEVERE CALORIC DEFICIT

Do not attempt to reduce your caloric intake during the first few days. Eat the same quantity of food you usually eat while changing the macro composition: fewer carbs, moderate protein, and more fat.

6. TAKE IT EASY WITH EXERCISE

Reduce the volume and intensity of exercise for the first few days (and maybe even during the first few weeks) to reduce the added stressors and promote a favorable transition. Focus on lighter activities like yoga and leisurely swims or walks.

PHASE 2: TRANSITIONING TO FAT-BURNING MODE

In phase 2, your body will start to transition to effectively using fat and ketones for fuel. This will result in higher feelings of fullness throughout the day, stable blood sugar levels, fewer cravings, endless energy, better mood, laser-sharp focus, etc. This will start at the end of the first week and last for another six to eight weeks, depending on your adherence and prior metabolic health.

1. CONTINUE TO REPLENISH ELECTROLYTES

Don't skimp on your electrolytes. It's essential to continue replenishing these minerals (primarily sodium, magnesium, and potassium) every day, especially surrounding physical activity.

2. EXTEND YOUR FASTING WINDOW

Now that your blood sugar is beginning to stabilize and you're starting to feel more satiated during the day, try to reduce snacking, extend your morning fast, and shut the kitchen down earlier at night.

3. REDUCE CALORIC INTAKE FOR FAT LOSS

As you become efficient at using fat and ketones for fuel while feeling more satiated during the day, you should naturally decrease the amount of food you're consuming. This will allow you to start burning excess body fat. Use the guidelines (Macronutrient Ratios for Weight Loss) as a starting place and adjust accordingly.

4. DON'T CHASE KETONES

If you regularly test ketones, you may start to reduce your urine or blood levels. This is because your body and cells are starting to become more efficient at using fatty acids and ketones for fuel, which is a good thing! See here for more details on testing ketones.

PHASE 3: BECOMING METABOLICALLY FLEXIBLE/ EFFICIENT

Once this is achieved, usually after four to six months or even up to a year, most people can effectively maintain a low-carbohydrate lifestyle while incorporating healthy carb sources and enjoying occasional indulgences.

1. KNOW THAT THIS IS NOT A DIET, RATHER A LIFESTYLE

If you look at Keto as a diet, you will not succeed in the long term. If you go back to what you were doing before, you will end up exactly where you started.

2. EXPERIMENT WITH SMALL INCREASES IN PROTEIN AND CARBS

After you've completely transitioned from a sugar burner to a fat-burner, you can start to play around with your protein and carb threshold. Some people can bump up their carb and protein intake while remaining in ketosis.

3. EASE OF GOING IN AND OUT OF KETOSIS

Now that you're a thriving fat-burner, your body will give you a bit more leeway when it comes to indulging in some carbs every once in a while. But don't use this as an excuse to eat a whole carton of ice cream.

Side Effects during the Keto Diet and How to Overcome Them

The Keto diet is quite simple, just eat 75% fats, 20% protein, and 5% carbs. It is a general practice, most ketogenic beginners follow, and they maintain their body quite quickly. However, when you cross the age of 50, there are many challenges which you have to go through. Below is the list of those challenges, along with their solutions.

KETO-FLU

An abrupt shift of diet, from the regular intake of carbs to a limited amount, can cause Keto-flu, also known as carb withdrawal. It usually occurs after one to two days of withdrawal. Its symptoms include headache, muscle soreness, poor focus, sugar cravings, brain fog, irritability, insomnia, or weakness. The body will take some time for it to jump from burning carbohydrates to burning fats. Therefore, an abrupt transformation of diet sends your body into starvation mode, giving you those unpleasant symptoms.

Solution:

- Stay well, hydrated.

- Electrolytes Supplementation.

- Consume More Healthy Fats.

- Consume exogenous Ketone Supplement.

MUSCLE CRAMPS AND DEHYDRATION

Carbs need water for their storage, unlike fats. Hence, instead of being retained, a smaller amount of water is stored during the Keto diet, and the kidneys excrete more amount of sodium. Due to this, you can quickly get dehydrated while on the Keto diet, especially at the beginning. Due to this condition, low electrolyte concentration and dehydration, muscle cramping is inevitable.

Solution:

- Consult your doctor and complain to him/her about the problems you are facing.

- Add electrolytes supplements three major electrolytes, such as potassium, sodium, and magnesium.

- Ensure drinking a lot of water to remain hydrated.

INSOMNIA

Although there is not any research that has shown the effect of a Keto diet on sleep deprivation, there some people who have complained about a lack of quality sleep during the Keto diet. If this is the case with you, then once in a while, eating some high–quality carbs before bed can prove to be of enormous help.

Solution:

Before sleeping, take one teaspoon of raw honey. This will give your body adequate high-quality carbs during your sleep.

BRAIN FOG

When you eat fewer carbs, your body demands it; "I am hungry, and I want something to eat." When its wish isn't accommodated, it makes you fuzzy-headed. This is the brain's way of demanding more glucose. Because, up until now, that's the only fuel it has ever known.

Solution:

The best solution to remedy this condition is to ignore it and keep eating fat only. Ultimately, your brain will adapt to its new fuel, and your head will become more apparent than ever before.

CONSTIPATION

Consuming carbs lesser than 20g of per day means insufficient fibers, which ultimately results in constipation and irritable bowel syndrome. Constipation also occurs when you are not drinking enough water. The following are some remedies to aid you in your constipation.

Solution:

- Add leafy and good vegetables to your diet.

- Try cyclical Keto from time to time.

- Add enough natural salt such as Himalayan pink salt to your diet.

- Always remain hydrated and take electrolyte supplements.

- Do exercise regularly; it will also help you in relieving constipation problems.

- Try to take the recommended dosage of a good-quality digestive enzyme before or after every meal.

- Consume psyllium husk every morning. Mix one teaspoon in 1/2 cup of water and let it sit for 1 minute before drinking.

DIARRHEA

Some people have diarrhea difficulties while on the Keto diet. Your body may react this way because of an increasing amount of fat intake, as it isn't yet able to produce and store enough bile to break down all the fat you're eating.

Solution:

- Reduce the amount of fat you're eating by at least 10 percent.

- Simultaneously, increase the number of fermented foods in your diets such as kombucha, water kefir, sauerkraut, kimchi, or your favorite fermented vegetable.

- Add apple cider vinegar to your drinks and salad dressings.

- Consider trying an ox bile supplement.

- To cure diarrhea, lower your fat intake for seven days—or until you have adapted to the new changes. Then, gradually increase your fat intake back up to where it was.

KETO RASH

Keto rash, also called prurigo pigmentosa, is an itchy red rash that can develop on the neck, chest, back, and armpit areas; it is neither dangerous nor life-threatening. Although very rare, it sometimes occurs when people follow a strict ketogenic diet, usually 80 percent fat or higher. Other causative agents are hormonal imbalances, allergen exposure, and gut bacteria.

Solution:

- Support your skin with adequate supplements and anti-inflammatory foods such as DHA, omega- 3 supplements, or turmeric latte.

- Keep yourself away from irritants like heat, sweat, or friction.

- Reintroduce some carbs in your diet, though avoid consuming a lot of bread.

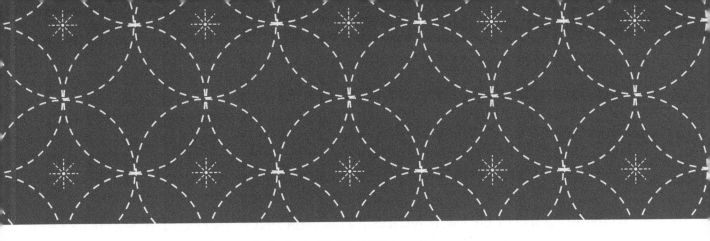

CHAPTER 4
COMMON MISTAKES AND HOW TO AVOID THEM

Let's now introduce the concept of ketosis: Ketosis is a condition in which the body obtains energy by burning fat and producing so-called ketones. Typically, this situation occurs when blood glucose levels rise due to a decrease in insulin. Low ketosis levels are normal, but when ketones increase a lot in a short time, they can also have serious adverse effects.

That is, ketosis is the condition that we must achieve. It is our final result, the reason why we started the ketogenic diet. Knowing this new concept, let's see what the main errors in the ketogenic diet are.

GIVE UP BEFORE COMPLETING KETOSIS

Nutritional ketosis is a mandatory step and brings more or less evident and more or less long aftermath. These vary based on how much carbohydrate has been abused previously and how much our liver is overloaded.

While the body is moving from burning sugar to burning fat, we have the sensation of feeling "poisoned" and "weighed down."

They are the toxins that are rising and, time a week or two, and it starts to bloom again.

Other symptoms related to the ketosis that is taking place are:

- Bad breath

- Slight nausea

- An initial hunger for sugars

- Tiredness

- Nervousness

- A slight sadness

These latter symptoms are linked to the impact that the elimination of sugars and carbohydrates has on our mind, which, by stimulating the same opiate receptors, make us feel happy and satisfied.

Now by stopping them and losing this stimulus, it may happen that, on the contrary, we feel a little sad and nervous.

Many are frightened of these symptoms and not being well informed. They believe that the ketogenic diet is not for them, that they are worse than when they started and abandon everything before going all the way to ketosis.

RUNNING INTO DEFICIENCIES IN SALTS AND MINERALS

A possible lack of minerals can exacerbate the desire for sugars that are accused at the beginning. It is, therefore, necessary to integrate with the right doses of potassium, magnesium, and sodium. Using Himalayan salt, eating salty snacks, using magnesium in the evening could be just as many ways to remedy this mistake.

CONSUME TOO MUCH PROTEIN

Higher doses of protein help overcome hunger crises, but it is good to go back to consuming the right amount.

To find out how many proteins to consume, just multiply your body weight by 0.8 (if you make a regular physical effort) or 1.2 (if you are a sportsman).

Another common mistake is to consume poor-quality proteins, such as pork and cold cuts.

INSUFFICIENT FAT CONSUMPTION

This is another mistake that is easy to run into if we follow the ketogenic diet. We continue to be afraid of consuming fats and not using all-natural sources: coconut oil, ghee, MCT oil, egg yolk, and fatty fish, and butter, avocado. The opposite mistake is to exaggerate with oilseeds: walnuts, almonds, flax seeds, pumpkin seeds. If we neglect to soak in advance with water and lemon, we also absorb the physic acid they contain, a pro substance inflammatory and antinutrient.

CONSUME BAD QUALITY FOOD

It is another of the most common mistakes. We focus on weight loss, but continue to consume frozen, canned, highly processed food and, as mentioned, proteins that are practical and quick to eat but of low quality.

DO NOT INTRODUCE THE RIGHT AMOUNT OF FIBER

Vegetables should always be fresh, consumed in twice the amount of protein, and always cooked intelligently, never subjected to overcooking or too high temperatures.

In everyday life, if present, however, we often resort to ready-made, frozen, or packaged vegetables.

Also, concerning fruit, we often resort to the very sugary ones; we forget that there are many berries with a low glycemic index: berries, mulberries, goji berries, Inca berries, maqui.

EAT RAW VEGETABLES

I know this may surprise you, but consuming large quantities of raw vegetables, centrifuged, cold smoothies, over time slow down digestion, cool it, undermine our ability to transform food and absorb nutrients. Over time, this exposes us to inevitable deficiencies: joint pain, teeth, nails and weak hair, anemia, tiredness, abnormal weight loss.

CONSUME THE HIGHEST PROTEIN LOAD AT DINNER

This is a mistake that involuntarily, we all commit. The work, the thousand commitments, leads us to stay out all day, to eat a frugal meal for lunch, or even not to consume it at all. Here the dinner turns into the only moment of the day in which we find our family members. We have more time, we are more relaxed, and we finally allow ourselves a real meal complete with vegetables, proteins, sometimes even carbohydrates, and then fruit or dessert to finish.

It escapes us that even the healthiest protein, the freshest or most organic food, weighs down the liver. During the night, this being busy helping digestion, it cannot perform the other precious task: to purify the blood, prepare hormones, energy for the next day.

NOT DRINKING ENOUGH

And above all, don't drink hot water. You got it right. Drinking hot water is another story entirely, a massive difference from drinking it even at room temperature. The benefits are many: more excellent digestibility and absorption, deep hydration of cells, brighter skin and hair, retention disappear, cellulite improves, kidneys are strengthened, digestion improves, and heartburn subsides.

So, in conclusion, if you avoid these nine mistakes:

- Give up before completing ketosis

- Incurring deficiencies in salts and minerals

- Consuming too much protein

- Consume few fats

- Consume lousy quality food

- Do not introduce the right amount of fiber

- Consume raw vegetables

- Introduce the highest protein load in the evening

- Do not drink incredibly hot water

That is, to allow the body to enter and exit the state of ketosis, to use fats as energy fuel, but also to burn glucose when we have it available.

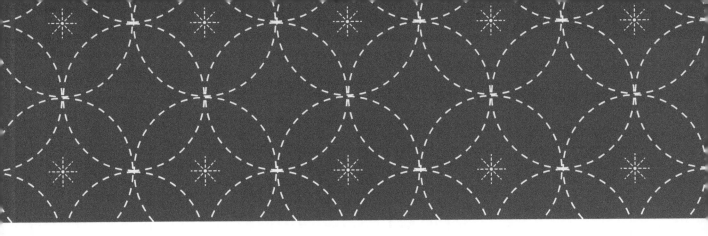

CHAPTER 5
21-DAY KETO MEAL PLAN

Day	Breakfast	Lunch	Snack	Dinner
1	Sesame Keto Bagels	Thai Cucumber Noodle Salad	Delicious Coffee Ice Cream	Creamy Garlic Chicken
2	Breakfast Omelet with Mushrooms	Chicken Quesadillas	Cute Peanut Balls	Turkey-Pepper Mix
3	Morning Coffee with Cream	Avocado Taco	Raspberry Mousse	Chicken Pan with Veggies and Pesto
4	Morning Coconut Porridge	Shrimp Lettuce Wraps with Buffalo Sauce	Chocolate Mug Muffin	Cabbage Soup with Beef
5	Spicy Cream Cheese Pancakes	Creamy Cauliflower Soup	Creamy Hot Chocolate	Shrimp Scampi with Garlic

6	Dairy-Free Pizza	Fatty Burger Bombs	Sugar-Free Lemon Bars	Fresh Avocado Soup
7	Baked Eggs in Avocado Halves	Salmon Sushi Rolls	Fatty Bombs with Cinnamon and Cardamom	Chinese Pork Bowl
8	Bracing Ginger Smoothie	Hearty Lunch Salad with Broccoli and Bacon	Quick and Simple Brownie	Cauliflower Cheesecake
9	Morning Coconut Porridge	Poke Bowl with Salmon and Veggies	Raspberry Mousse	Chicken Pan with Veggies and Pesto
10	Breakfast Omelet with Mushrooms	Wrapped Bacon Cheeseburger	Chocolate Spread with Hazelnuts	Quick Pumpkin Soup
11	Baked Eggs in Avocado Halves	Creamy Cauliflower Soup	Sugar-Free Lemon Bars	Simple Tuna Salad
12	Morning Coffee with Cream	Fatty Burger Bombs	Cute Peanut Balls	Cauliflower Rice Soup with Chicken
13	Spicy Cream Cheese Pancakes	Mediterranean Salad with Grilled Chicken	Chocolate Mug Muffin	Turkey-Pepper Mix
14	Sesame Keto Bagels	Chicken Quesadillas	Delicious Coffee Ice Cream	Shrimp Scampi with Garlic

15	Breakfast Omelet with Mushrooms	Avocado Taco	Fatty Bombs with Cinnamon and Cardamom	Cabbage Soup with Beef
16	Bracing Ginger Smoothie	Shrimp Lettuce Wraps with Buffalo Sauce	Quick and Simple Brownie	Chinese Pork Bowl
17	Dairy-Free Pizza	Thai Cucumber Noodle Salad	Creamy Hot Chocolate	Creamy Garlic Chicken
18	Morning Coconut Porridge	Salmon Sushi Rolls	Raspberry Mousse	Shrimp Scampi with Garlic
19	Morning Coffee with Cream	Poke Bowl with Salmon and Veggies	Chocolate Mug Muffin	Turkey-Pepper Mix
20	Baked Eggs in Avocado Halves	Hearty Lunch Salad with Broccoli and Bacon	Sugar-Free Lemon Bars	Chicken Pan with Veggies and Pesto
21	Spicy Cream Cheese Pancakes	Fatty Burger Bombs	Cute Peanut Balls	Cauliflower Cheesecake

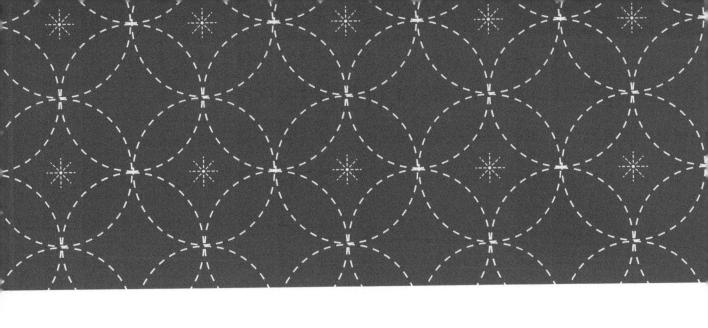

CHAPTER 6
BREAKFAST

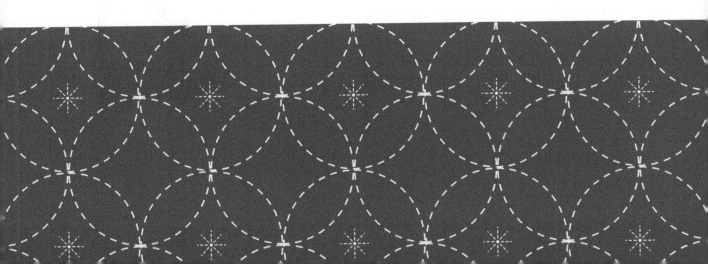

1. BACON & EGG BREAKFAST MUFFINS

INGREDIENTS

- 8 large Eggs
- 8 slices Bacon
- .66 cup Green onion

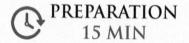 **PREPARATION** 15 MIN 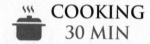 **COOKING** 30 MIN 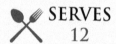 **SERVES** 12

DIRECTIONS

1. Warm the oven at 350° Fahrenheit. Spritz the muffin tin wells using a cooking oil spray. Chop the onions and set them aside.
2. Prepare a large skillet using the medium temperature setting. Fry the bacon until it's crispy and place on a layer of paper towels to drain the grease. Chop it into small pieces after it has cooled.
3. Whisk the eggs, bacon, and green onions, mixing well until all of the ingredients are incorporated. Dump the egg mixture into the muffin tin (halfway full). Bake it for about 20 to 25 minutes. Cool slightly and serve.

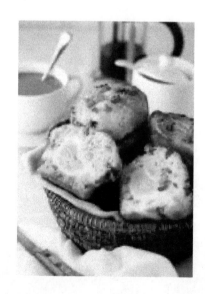

Nutritions:

Carbohydrates: 0.4 g

Protein: 5.6 g

Fats: 4.9 g

Calories: 69 kcal

2. BACON HASH

INGREDIENTS

- 1 Small green pepper
- 2 Jalapenos
- 1 Small onion
- 4 Eggs
- 6 Bacon slices

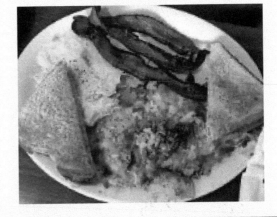

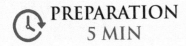 **PREPARATION** 5 MIN

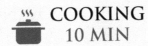 **COOKING** 10 MIN

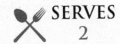 **SERVES** 2

DIRECTIONS

1. Chop the bacon into chunks using a food processor. Set aside for now. Slice the peppers and onions into thin strips. Dice the jalapenos as small as possible.
2. Heat a skillet and fry the veggies. Once browned, combine the ingredients and cook until crispy. Place on a serving dish with the eggs.

Nutritions:

Carbohydrates: 9 g
Protein: 23 g

Fats: 24 g
Calories: 366 kcal

3. BAGELS WITH CHEESE

INGREDIENTS

- 2.5 cups Mozzarella cheese
- 1 tsp. Baking powder
- 3 oz Cream cheese
- 1.5 cups Almond flour
- 2 Eggs

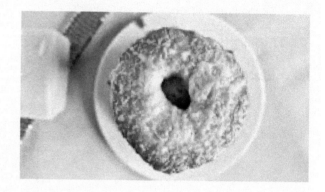

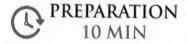 **PREPARATION**
10 MIN

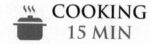 **COOKING**
15 MIN

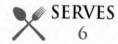 **SERVES**
6

DIRECTIONS

1. Shred the mozzarella and combine with the flour, baking powder, and cream cheese in a mixing container. Pop into the microwave for about one minute. Mix well.
2. Let the mixture cool and add the eggs. Break apart into six sections and shape into round bagels. Note: You can also sprinkle with a seasoning of your choice or pinch of salt if desired.
3. Bake for approximately 12 minutes. Serve or cool and store.

Nutritions:

Carbohydrates: 8 g
Protein: 19 g

Fats: 31 g
Calories: 374 kcal

4. BAKED APPLES

INGREDIENTS

- 4 tsp Keto-friendly sweetener
- 75 tsp Cinnamon
- .25 cup chopped pecans
- 4 large Granny Smith apples

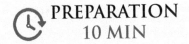 **PREPARATION**
10 MIN

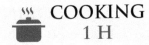 **COOKING**
1 H

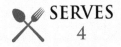 **SERVES**
4

DIRECTIONS

1. Set the oven temperature at 375° Fahrenheit. Mix the sweetener with the cinnamon and pecans. Core the apple and add the prepared stuffing.
2. Add enough water into the baking dish to cover the bottom of the apple. Bake them for about 45 minutes to 1 hour.

Nutritions:

Carbohydrates: 16 g
Protein: 6.8 g

Fats: 19.9 g
Calories: 175 kcal

5. BAKED EGGS IN THE AVOCADO

INGREDIENTS

- Half of 1 Avocado
- 1 Egg
- 1 tbsp Olive oil
- Half cup shredded cheddar cheese

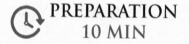 **PREPARATION**
10 MIN

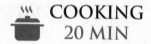 **COOKING**
20 MIN

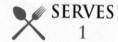 **SERVES**
1

DIRECTIONS

1. Heat the oven to reach 425° Fahrenheit.
2. Discard the avocado pit and remove just enough of the 'insides' to add the egg. Drizzle with oil and break the egg into the shell.
3. Sprinkle with cheese and bake them for 15 to 16 minutes until the egg is the way you prefer. Serve.

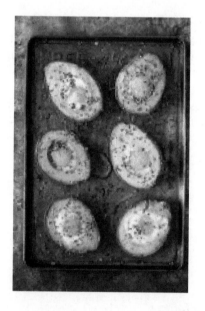

Nutritions:

Carbohydrates: 3 g
Protein: 21 g

Fats: 52 g
Calories: 452 kcal

6. BANANA PANCAKES

INGREDIENTS

- Butter
- 2 Bananas
- 4 Eggs
- 1 tsp Cinnamon
- 1 tsp Baking powder (Optional)

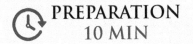 **PREPARATION**
10 MIN

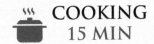 **COOKING**
15 MIN

 **SERVES**
3

DIRECTIONS

1. Combine each of the ingredients. Melt a portion of butter in a skillet using the medium temperature setting.
2. Prepare the pancakes 1-2 minutes per side. Cook them with the lid on for the first part of the cooking cycle for a fluffier pancake.
3. Serve plain or with your favorite garnishes such as a dollop of coconut cream or fresh berries.

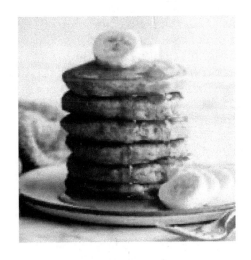

Nutritions:

Carbohydrates: 6.8 g
Total Fat: 7 g

Calories: 157 kcal

7. BREAKFAST SKILLET

INGREDIENTS

- 1 lb. Organic ground turkey/grass-fed beef
- 6 Organic eggs
- 1 cup Keto-friendly salsa of choice

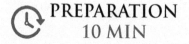 **PREPARATION**
10 MIN

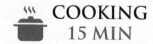 **COOKING**
15 MIN

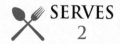 **SERVES**
2

DIRECTIONS

1. Warm the skillet using oil (medium heat). Add the turkey and simmer until the pink is gone. Fold in the salsa and simmer for two to three minutes.
2. Crack the eggs and add to the top of the turkey base. Place a lid on the pot and cook for seven minutes until the whites of the eggs are opaque.
3. Note: The cooking time will vary depending on how you like the eggs prepared

Nutritions:

Carbohydrates: 7.1 g
Protein: 65.2 g

Fats: 32 g
Calories: 5 kcal

8. GREEN BANANA PANCAKES

INGREDIENTS

- 2 large peeled bananas
- 2 eggs
- 6 tablespoons coconut flour
- 2 teaspoons cassava flour or arrowroot starch
- Pinch salt
- ¼ teaspoon stevia powder
- 1 tablespoon baking powder
- Coconut oil or grass-fed butter

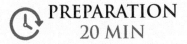 **PREPARATION**
20 MIN

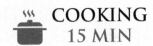 **COOKING**
15 MIN

 **SERVES**
4

DIRECTIONS

1. Puree the banana until smooth.
2. Mix the coconut flour, stevia, arrowroot or cassava, baking soda, and a pinch of salt in a mixing bowl to make a powder form.
3. Whisk egg very lightly in a small bowl, then pour into the banana, mix well.
4. Then add in the powder mixture in it. If the mixture is too thick, add some water with a spoon to make it slightly thin; do not overwater.
5. Preheat a skillet along with butter, ghee, or oil.
6. Pour in the batter in the skillet with a spoon.
7. When it is golden brown from the top, flip it, cook until brown, and take it out on a plate. Serve hot.

Nutritions:

Calories 224 kcal
Cholesterol 224 mg

Total Fat 32g
Total Carbs 5g

9. BERRY BREAD SPREAD

INGREDIENTS

- 2 cups coconut cream
- 2 ounces strawberries
- 1 ½ ounce blueberries
- 1 ½ ounce raspberries
- ½ teaspoon coconut extract

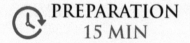 **PREPARATION**
15 MIN

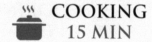 **COOKING**
15 MIN

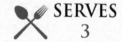 **SERVES**
3

DIRECTIONS

1. Dice three of each berry in small pieces separately.
2. Blend the remaining strawberries, blueberries, and raspberries in a blender until smooth.
3. Mix in the coconut extract and coconut cream.
4. Blend again until smooth, then add in the diced berries.
5. Serve chilled.

Nutritions:

Calories: 285 kcal
Total Fat: 18 g

Total Carbs: 5.5 g
Protein: 6.8 g

10. CHOCOLATE BREAD SPREAD

INGREDIENTS

- 4 cups sweet cream
- 2 ounces coconut oil
- 3 ounces chocolate
- 1 teaspoon coconut extract
- 1 tablespoon powdered cacao
- Groundnuts [optional]

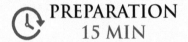 **PREPARATION**
15 MIN

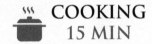 **COOKING**
15 MIN

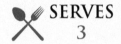 **SERVES**
3

DIRECTIONS

1. Put sweet cream in a microwavable bowl and heat for 10-15 seconds
2. Add in coconut oil and mix, then mix in the chocolate and powdered cacao, mix well.
3. Heat the mixture in the microwave for a minute or so.
4. When it is warm, add groundnuts, if desired.
5. Pour in fridge bowls, and chill.
6. Serve as you desire.

Nutritions:

Calories: 257 kcal
Total Fat: 19 g

Total Carbs:7.5 g
Protein: 11.8 g

11. KETO ALMOND CEREAL

INGREDIENTS

- 3 cups unsweetened coconut flakes
- 1 cup sliced almonds
- ¾ tablespoon cinnamon
- ¾ tablespoon nutmeg

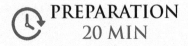 **PREPARATION** 20 MIN

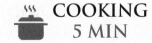 **COOKING** 5 MIN

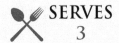 **SERVES** 3

DIRECTIONS

1. Preheat oven to 250 degrees F.
2. Mix the almonds and coconut flakes together, then add nutmeg and cinnamon. Mix well.
3. Spread the nut mixture on a baking tray, and bake for 3-5 minutes.
4. Take out, when slightly brown.
5. Enjoy with milk.

Nutritions:

Calories: 104 kcal   Carbohydrates: 4 g
Fat: 15 g   Protein: 5 g

12. KETO GRANOLA CEREAL

INGREDIENTS

- 1 cup flaxseeds
- 1 large egg
- 1 cup Almonds
- 1 cup Hazelnuts
- 1 cup Pecans
- 1/3 cup Pumpkin seeds
- 1/3 cup Sunflower seeds
- 1/4 cup melted butter/ coconut oil/ ghee for dairy-free
- 1 tsp Vanilla extract

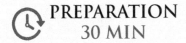 **PREPARATION** 30 MIN

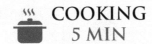 **COOKING** 5 MIN

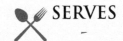 **SERVES** -

DIRECTIONS

1. Preheat the oven to 370 degrees F, and line the baking tray with wax or parchment paper.
2. Pulse almonds and hazelnuts in a food processor intermittently, until chopped into large pieces, then add pecans and chop again into large pieces. Pecans are added later since they are softer.
3. Add the pumpkin seeds, sunflower seeds, and flaxseeds, and pulse just until everything is mixed well. Don't over-process; you should have most seeds in intact form.
4. Whisk an egg white and pour it into the food processor.
5. Then, whisk together the melted butter and vanilla extract in a small bowl, and evenly pour that in the food processor, too.
6. Pulse again to mix well until it combines in the form of coarse meal and nut pieces, and everything should be a little moist from the egg white and butter.
7. Transfer the mixture to the baking tray, evenly pressing, bake for 15 to 18 minutes, or until slightly brown from the edges.
8. Let it cool,
9. Break it into pieces.

Nutritions:

Calories 441 kcal
Fat: 40 g

Carbohydrates: 4 g
Protein: 16 g

13. SESAME KETO BAGELS

INGREDIENTS

- 2 cups almond flour
- 3 eggs
- 1 Tbsp baking powder
- 2½ cups Mozzarella cheese, shredded
- ½ cream cheese, cubed
- 1 pinch salt
- 2-3 tsp sesame seeds

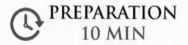 **PREPARATION**
10 MIN

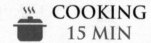 **COOKING**
15 MIN

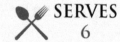 **SERVES**
6

DIRECTIONS

1. Preheat the oven to 425°F.
2. Use a medium bowl to whisk the almond flour and baking powder. Add the mozzarella cheese and cubed cream cheese into a large bowl, mix and microwave for 90 seconds. Place 2 eggs into the almond mixture and stir thoroughly to form a dough.
3. Part your dough into 6 portions and make it into balls. Press every dough ball slightly to make a hole in the center and put your ball on the baking mat.
4. Brush the top of every bagel with the remaining egg and top with sesame seeds.
5. Bake for about 15 minutes.

Nutritions:

Carbohydrates: 9 g
Fat: 39 g

Protein: 23 g
Calories: 469 kcal

14. BAKED EGGS IN AVOCADO HALVES

INGREDIENTS

- 1 large avocado
- 2 eggs
- 3 oz bacon
- 1 small tomato, chopped
- 1 pinch salt and paper
- ½ oz lettuce, shredded

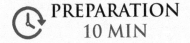 **PREPARATION** 10 MIN

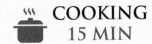 **COOKING** 15 MIN

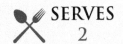 **SERVES** 2

DIRECTIONS

1. Fry the bacon and cut it. Put aside.
2. Warm your oven to 375°F.
3. Cut the avocado into two halves and make a large hole in each half to place the egg in it.
4. Put avocado halves onto a baking sheet, place eggs, add salt and pepper. Cover the eggs with chopped tomatoes and bacon.
5. Bake for 15 minutes and top your avocadoes with shredded lettuce at the end.

Nutritions:

Carbohydrates: 7 g
Fat: 72 g

Protein: 26 g
Calories: 810 kcal

15. SPICY CREAM CHEESE PANCAKES

INGREDIENTS

- 3 eggs
- 9 Tbsp cottage cheese
- Salt, to taste
- ½ Tbsp psyllium husk powder
- Butter, for frying
- 4 oz cream cheese
- 1 Tbsp green pesto
- 1 Tbsp olive oil
- ¼ red onion, finely sliced
- Black pepper, to taste

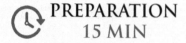 **PREPARATION**
15 MIN

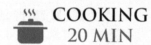 **COOKING**
20 MIN

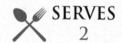 **SERVES**
2

DIRECTIONS

1. Combine cream cheese, olive oil, and pesto. Put this mixture aside.
2. Blend eggs, psyllium husk powder, cottage cheese, and salt until the mixture is smooth. Leave it for 5 minutes.
3. Heat the butter in the pan and put several dollops of cottage cheese batter into the pan. Fry for a few minutes each side.
4. Top your pancakes with a large amount of cream cheese mixture and several red onion slices.
5. Add black pepper and olive oil.

Nutritions:

Carbohydrates: 7 g
Fat: 38 g

Protein: 18 g
Calories: 449 kcal

16. BRACING GINGER SMOOTHIE

INGREDIENTS

- 1/3 cup coconut cream
- 2/3 cup water
- 2 Tbsp lime juice
- 1 oz spinach, frozen
- 2 Tbsp ginger, grated

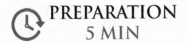 **PREPARATION**
5 MIN

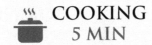 **COOKING**
5 MIN

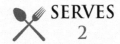 **SERVES**
2

DIRECTIONS

1. Blend all the ingredients. Add 1 Tbsp lime at first and increase the amount if necessary.
2. Top with grated ginger and enjoy your smoothie!

Nutritions:

Carbohydrates: 3 g
Fat: 8 g

Protein: 1 g
Calories: 82 kcal

17. MORNING COFFEE WITH CREAM

INGREDIENTS

- ¾ cup coffee
- ¼ cup whipping cream

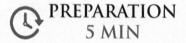 **PREPARATION**
5 MIN

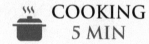 **COOKING**
5 MIN

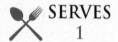 **SERVES**
1

DIRECTIONS

1. Make your favorite coffee.
2. Put heavy cream in a saucepan and heat slowly until you get a frothy texture.
3. Pour the hot cream into a big cup, add coffee and enjoy your morning drink.

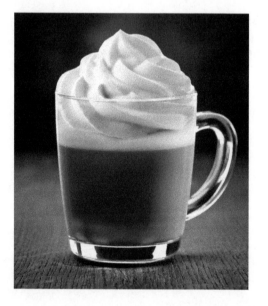

Nutritions:

Carbohydrates: 2 g
Fat: 21 g

Protein: 2 g
Calories: 202 kcal

18. EGG-CRUST PIZZA

INGREDIENTS

- ¼ teaspoon dried oregano to taste
- ½ teaspoon spike seasoning to taste
- 1 ounce mozzarella, chopped into small cubes
- 6 – 8 sliced thinly black olives
- 6 slices of turkey pepperoni, sliced into half
- 4-5 thinly sliced small grape tomatoes
- 2 eggs, beaten well
- 1-2 teaspoons olive oil

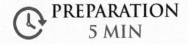 **PREPARATION** 5 MIN   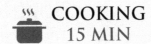 **COOKING** 15 MIN   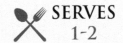 **SERVES** 1-2

DIRECTIONS

1. Preheat the broiler in an oven than in a small bowl, beat well the eggs. Cut the pepperoni and tomatoes in slices then cut the mozzarella cheese into cubes.
2. Put olive oil in a skillet over medium heat, then heat the pan for around one minute until it begins to get hot. Add in eggs and season with oregano and spike seasoning, then cook for around 2 minutes until the eggs begin to set at the bottom.
3. Drizzle half of the mozzarella, olives, pepperoni, and tomatoes on the eggs followed by another layer of the remaining half of the above ingredients. Ensure that there is a lot of cheese on the topmost layers. Cover the skillet using a lid and cook until the cheese begins to melt and the eggs are set, for around 3-4 minutes.
4. Place the pan under the preheated broiler and cook until the top has browned and the cheese has melted nicely for around 2-3 minutes. Serve immediately.

Nutritions:

Calories: 363 kcal
Fats: 24.1 g

Carbohydrates: 20.8 g
Proteins: 19.25 g

19. BREAKFAST ROLL-UPS

INGREDIENTS

- Non-stick cooking spray
- 5 patties cooked breakfast sausage
- 5 slices cooked bacon
- 1.5 cups cheddar cheese, shredded
- Pepper and salt
- 10 large eggs

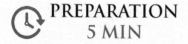 **PREPARATION** 5 MIN

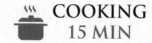 **COOKING** 15 MIN

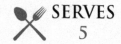 **SERVES** 5

DIRECTIONS

1. Heat a skillet on medium to high heat, then using a whisk, combine two of the eggs in a mixing bowl.
2. After the pan has become hot, lower the heat to medium-low heat then put in the eggs. If you want to, you can utilize some cooking spray.
3. Season eggs with some pepper and salt.
4. Cover eggs, leave them to cook for a couple of minutes or until the eggs are almost cooked.
5. Drizzle around 1/3 cup of cheese on top of the eggs, then place a strip of bacon and divide the sausage into two and place on top.
6. Roll the egg carefully on top of the fillings. The roll-up will almost look like a taquito. If you have a hard time folding over the egg, use a spatula to keep the egg intact until the egg has molded into a roll-up.
7. Put aside the roll-up then repeat the above steps until you have four more roll-ups; you should have 5 roll-ups in total.

Nutritions:

Calories: 412.2 kcal
Fats: 31.66 g
Carbohydrates: 2.26 g
Proteins: 28.21g

20. BASIC OPIE ROLLS

INGREDIENTS

- 1/8 teaspoon salt
- 1/8 teaspoon cream of tartar
- 3 ounces cream cheese
- 3 large eggs

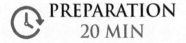 **PREPARATION**
20 MIN

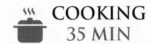 **COOKING**
35 MIN

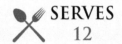 **SERVES**
12

DIRECTIONS

1. Preheat the oven to about 148.889 C or 300 degrees F, then separate the egg whites from egg yolks and place both eggs in different bowls. Using an electric mixer, beat well the egg whites until the mixture is very bubbly, then add in the cream of tartar and mix again until it forms a stiff peak.
2. In the bowl with the egg yolks, put in 3 ounces of cubed cheese and salt. Mix well until the mixture has doubled in size and is pale yellow. Put the egg white mixture into the egg yolk mixture then fold the mixture gently together.
3. Spray some oil on the cookie sheet coated with some parchment paper, then add dollops of the batter and bake for around 30 minutes.
4. When the upper part of the rolls is firm and golden they are ready. Leave them to cool for a few minutes on a wire rack. Enjoy with some coffee.

Nutritions:

Calories: 45 kcal
Fats: 4 g

Carbohydrates: 0 g
Proteins: 2 g

21. ALMOND COCONUT EGG WRAPS

INGREDIENTS

- 5 Organic eggs
- 1 tbsp Coconut flour
- 25 tsp Sea salt
- 2 tbsp almond meal

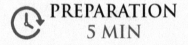 **PREPARATION**
5 MIN

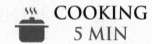 **COOKING**
5 MIN

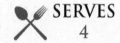 **SERVES**
4

DIRECTIONS

1. Combine the ingredients in a blender and work them until creamy. Heat a skillet using the med-high temperature setting.
2. Pour two tablespoons of batter into the skillet and cook - covered about three minutes. Turn it over to cook for another 3 minutes. Serve the wraps piping hot.

Nutritions:

Carbohydrates: 3 g
Protein: 8 g

Fats: 8 g
Calories: 111 kcal

22. BACON & AVOCADO OMELLETE

INGREDIENTS

- 1 slice Crispy bacon
- 2 large organic eggs
- 5 cup freshly grated parmesan cheese
- 2 tbsp Ghee or coconut oil or butter
- half of 1 small Avocado

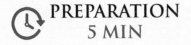 **PREPARATION**
5 MIN

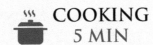 **COOKING**
5 MIN

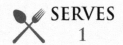 **SERVES**
1

DIRECTIONS

1. Prepare the bacon to your liking and set aside. Combine the eggs, parmesan cheese, and your choice of finely chopped herbs. Warm a skillet and add the butter/ghee to melt using the medium-high heat setting. When the pan is hot, whisk and add the eggs.

2. Prepare the omelet working it towards the middle of the pan for about 30 seconds. When firm, flip, and cook it for another 30 seconds. Arrange the omelet on a plate and garnish it with the crunched bacon bits. Serve with sliced avocado.

Nutritions:

Carbohydrates: 3.3 g
Protein: 30 g

Fats: 63 g
Calories: 719 kcal

23. BACON & CHEESE FRITTATA

INGREDIENTS

- 1 cup Heavy cream
- 6 Eggs
- 5 Crispy slices of bacon
- 2 Chopped green onions
- 4 oz Cheddar cheese
- Also Needed: 1 pie plate

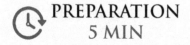 **PREPARATION**
5 MIN

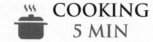 **COOKING**
5 MIN

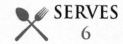 **SERVES**
6

DIRECTIONS

1. Warm the oven temperature to reach 350° Fahrenheit.
2. Whisk the eggs and seasonings. Empty into the pie pan and top off with the remainder of the ingredients. Bake 30-35 minutes. Wait for a few minutes before serving for best results.

Nutritions:

Carbohydrates: 2 g
Protein: 13 g

Fats: 29 g
Calories: 320 kcal

24. BACON AND EGG BREAKFAST SANDWICH

INGREDIENTS

- 2 cups bell peppers; chopped
- 1/2 tbsp. of avocado oil
- 3 eggs
- 4 bacon slices

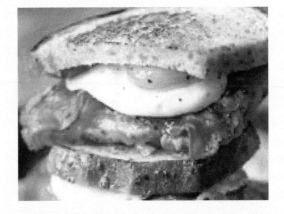

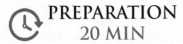 **PREPARATION**
20 MIN

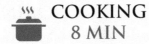 **COOKING**
8 MIN

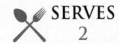 **SERVES**
2

DIRECTIONS

1. Heat up a pan with the oil over medium-high heat, add bell peppers, stir and cook until they are soft.
2. Heat up another pan over medium heat, add bacon, stir and cook until it's crispy.
3. In a bowl; whisk eggs really well and add them to bell peppers.
4. Cook until eggs are done for about 8 minutes. Divide half of the bacon slices between plates, add eggs, top with bacon slices, and serve.

Nutritions:

Calories: 200 kcal   Fiber: 3 g   Protein: 10 g
Fat: 4 g   Carbs: 6 g

25. KORMA CURRY

INGREDIENTS

- 3-pound chicken breast, skinless, boneless
- 1 teaspoon garam masala
- 1 teaspoon curry powder
- 1 tablespoon apple cider vinegar
- 1/2 cup coconut cream
- 1 cup organic almond milk
- 1 teaspoon ground coriander
- ¾ teaspoon ground cardamom
- 1/2 teaspoon ginger powder
- 1/4 teaspoon cayenne pepper
- ¾ teaspoon ground cinnamon

- 1 tomato, diced
- 1 teaspoon avocado oil
- 1/2 cup water

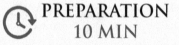 **PREPARATION** 10 MIN

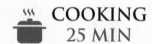 **COOKING** 25 MIN

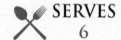 **SERVES** 6

DIRECTIONS

1. Chop the chicken breast and put it in the saucepan.
2. Add avocado oil and start to cook it over medium heat.
3. Sprinkle the chicken with garam masala, curry powder, apple cider vinegar, ground coriander, cardamom, ginger powder, cayenne pepper, ground cinnamon, and diced tomato. Mix up the ingredients carefully. Cook them for 10 minutes.
4. Add water, coconut cream, and almond milk. Sauté the meat for 10 minutes more.

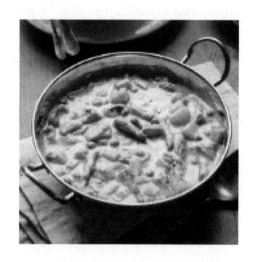

Nutritions:

Calories: 411 kcal
Fat: 19.3 g

Fiber: 0.9 g
Carbs: 6 g

Protein: 49.9 g

26. ZUCCHINI BARS

INGREDIENTS

- 3 zucchinis, grated
- 1/2 white onion, diced
- 2 teaspoons butter
- 3 eggs, whisked
- 4 tablespoons coconut flour
- 1 teaspoon salt
- 1/2 teaspoon ground black pepper
- 5 oz. goat cheese, crumbled
- 4 oz. Swiss cheese, shredded
- 1/2 cup spinach, chopped
- 1 teaspoon baking powder
- 1/2 teaspoon lemon juice

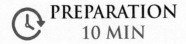 **PREPARATION** 10 MIN

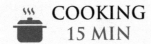 **COOKING** 15 MIN

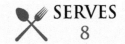 **SERVES** 8

DIRECTIONS

1. In the mixing bowl, mix up together grated zucchini, diced onion, eggs, coconut flour, salt, ground black pepper, crumbled cheese, chopped spinach, baking powder, and lemon juice.
2. Add butter and churn the mixture until homogenous.
3. Line the baking dish with baking paper.
4. Transfer the zucchini mixture into the baking dish and flatten it.
5. Preheat the oven to 365F and put the dish inside.
6. Cook it for 15 minutes. Then chill the meal well.
7. Cut it into bars.

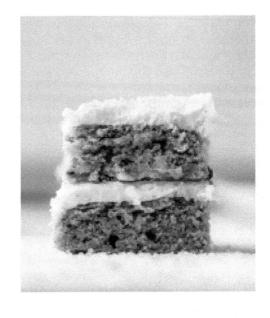

Nutritions:

Calories: 199 kcal
Fat: 1316 g

Fiber: 215 g
Carbs: 7.1 g

Protein: 13.1 g

27. MUSHROOM SOUP

INGREDIENTS

- 1 cup water
- 1 cup coconut milk
- 1 cup white mushrooms, chopped
- 1/2 carrot, chopped
- 1/4 white onion, diced
- 1 tablespoon butter
- 2 oz. turnip, chopped
- 1 teaspoon dried dill
- 1/2 teaspoon ground black pepper
- ¾ teaspoon smoked paprika
- 1 oz. celery stalk, chopped

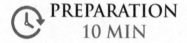 **PREPARATION** 10 MIN
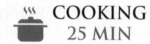 **COOKING** 25 MIN
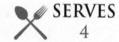 **SERVES** 4

DIRECTIONS

1. Pour water and coconut milk into the saucepan. Bring the liquid to a boil.
2. Add chopped mushrooms, carrots, and turnip. Close the lid and boil for 10 minutes.
3. Meanwhile, put butter in the skillet. Add diced onion. Sprinkle it with dill, ground black pepper, and smoked paprika. Roast the onion for 3 minutes.
4. Add the roasted onion in the soup mixture.
5. Then add chopped celery stalk. Close the lid.
6. Cook soup for 10 minutes.
7. Then ladle it into the serving bowls.

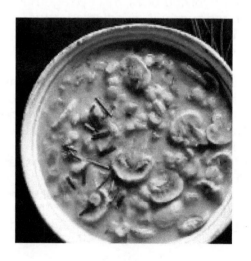

Nutritions:

Calories: 181 kcal
Fat: 17.3 g

Fiber: 2.5 g
Carbs: 6.9 g

Protein: 2.4 g

28. STUFFED PORTOBELLO MUSHROOMS

INGREDIENTS

- 2 Portobello mushrooms
- 1 cup spinach, chopped, steamed
- 2 oz. artichoke hearts, drained, chopped
- 1 tablespoon coconut cream
- 1 tablespoon cream cheese
- 1 teaspoon minced garlic
- 1 tablespoon fresh cilantro, chopped
- 3 oz. Cheddar cheese, grated
- 1/2 teaspoon ground black pepper
- 2 tablespoons olive oil
- 1/2 teaspoon salt

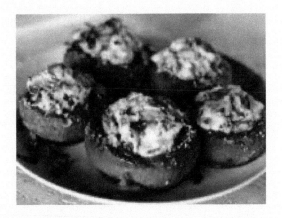

PREPARATION 10 MIN	COOKING 10 MIN	SERVES 4

DIRECTIONS

1. Sprinkle mushrooms with olive oil and place them in the tray.
2. Transfer the tray to the preheated 360°F oven and broil them for 5 minutes.
3. Meanwhile, blend together artichoke hearts, coconut cream, cream cheese, minced garlic, and chopped cilantro.
4. Add grated cheese in the mixture and sprinkle with ground black pepper and salt.
5. Fill the broiled mushrooms with the cheese mixture and cook them for 5 minutes more. Serve the mushrooms only hot.

Nutritions:

Calories: 183 kcal
Fat: 16.3 g

Fiber: 1.9 g
Carbs: 3 g

Protein: 7.7 g

29. LETTUCE SALAD

INGREDIENTS

- 1 cup Romaine lettuce, roughly chopped
- 3 oz. seitan, chopped
- 1 tablespoon avocado oil
- 1 teaspoon sunflower seeds
- 1 teaspoon lemon juice
- 1 egg, boiled, peeled
- 2 oz. Cheddar of cheese, shredded

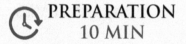 **PREPARATION**
10 MIN

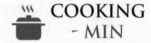 **COOKING**
- MIN

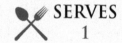 **SERVES**
1

DIRECTIONS

1. Place lettuce in the salad bowl. Add chopped seitan and shredded cheese.
2. Then chop the egg roughly and add it in the salad bowl too.
3. Mix up together lemon juice with the avocado oil.
4. Sprinkle the salad with the oil mixture and sunflower seeds. Don't stir the salad before serving.

Nutritions:

Calories: 663 kcal
Fat: 29.5 g

Fiber: 4.7 g
Carbs: 3.8 g

Protein: 84.2 g

30. ONION SOUP

INGREDIENTS

- 2 cups white onion, diced
- 4 tablespoon butter
- 1/2 cup white mushrooms, chopped
- 3 cups water
- 1 cup heavy cream
- 1 teaspoon salt
- 1 teaspoon chili flakes
- 1 teaspoon garlic powder

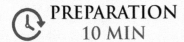 **PREPARATION**
10 MIN

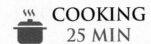 **COOKING**
25 MIN

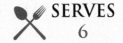 **SERVES**
6

DIRECTIONS

1. Put butter in the saucepan and melt it.
2. Add diced white onion, chili flakes, and garlic powder. Mix it up and sauté for 10 minutes over medium-low heat.
3. Then add water, heavy cream, and chopped mushrooms. Close the lid.
4. Cook the soup for 15 minutes more.
5. Then blend the soup until you get the creamy texture. Ladle it in the bowls.

Nutritions:

Calories: 155 kcal
Fat: 15.1 g

Fiber: 0.9 g
Carbs: 4.7 g

Protein: 1.2 g

31. ASPARAGUS SALAD

INGREDIENTS

- 10 oz. asparagus
- 1 tablespoon olive oil
- 1/2 teaspoon white pepper
- 4 oz. Feta cheese, crumbled
- 1 cup lettuce, chopped
- 1 tablespoon canola oil
- 1 teaspoon apple cider vinegar
- 1 tomato, diced

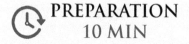 **PREPARATION**
10 MIN

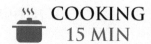 **COOKING**
15 MIN

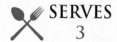 **SERVES**
3

DIRECTIONS

1. Preheat the oven to 365F.
2. Place asparagus in the tray, sprinkle with olive oil and white pepper and transfer to the preheated oven. Cook it for 15 minutes.
3. Meanwhile, put crumbled Feta in the salad bowl.
4. Add chopped lettuce and diced tomato.
5. Sprinkle the ingredients with apple cider vinegar.
6. Chill the cooked asparagus to the room temperature and add in the salad.
7. Shake the salad gently before serving.

Nutritions:

Calories: 207 kcal   Fiber: 2.4 g   Protein: 7.8 g
Fat : 17.6 g   Carbs: 6.8 g

32. CHEESY BREAKFAST MUFFINS

INGREDIENTS

- 4 tablespoons melted butter
- 3/4 tablespoon baking powder
- 1 cup almond flour
- 2 large eggs, lightly beaten
- 2 ounces cream cheese mixed with 2 tablespoons heavy whipping cream
- A handful of shredded Mexican blend cheese

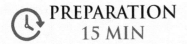 **PREPARATION** 15 MIN

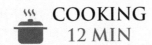 **COOKING** 12 MIN

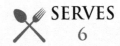 **SERVES** 6

DIRECTIONS

1. Preheat the oven to 400°F. Grease 6 muffin tin cups with melted butter and set aside.
2. Combine the baking powder and almond flour in a bowl. Stir well and set aside.
3. Stir together four tablespoons melted butter, eggs, shredded cheese, and cream cheese in a separate bowl.
4. The egg and the dry mixture must be combined using a hand mixer to beat until it is creamy and well blended.
5. The mixture must be scooped into the greased muffin cups evenly.
6. Baking time: 12 minutes

Nutritions:

Calories: 214 kcal
Fat: 15.6 g

Fiber: 3.1 g
Carbohydrates: 5.1 g

Protein: 9.5 g

33. SPINACH, MUSHROOM, AND GOAT CHEESE FRITTATA

INGREDIENTS

- 2 tablespoons olive oil
- 1 cup fresh mushrooms, sliced
- 6 bacon slices, cooked and chopped
- 1 cup spinach, shredded
- 10 large eggs, beaten
- 1/2 cup goat cheese, crumbled
- Pepper and salt

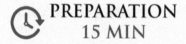 **PREPARATION** 15 MIN

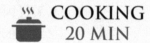 **COOKING** 20 MIN

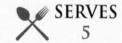 **SERVES** 5

DIRECTIONS

1. Preheat the oven to 350°F.
2. Heat oil and add the mushrooms and fry for 3 minutes until they start to brown, stirring frequently.
3. Fold in the bacon and spinach and cook for about 1 to 2 minutes, or until the spinach is wilted.
4. Slowly pour in the beaten eggs and cook for 3 to 4 minutes. Making use of a spatula, lift the edges for allowing uncooked egg to flow underneath.
5. Top with the goat cheese, and then sprinkle the salt and pepper to season.
6. Bake in the preheated oven for about 15 minutes until lightly golden brown around the edges.

Nutritions:

Calories: 265 kcal
Fat: 11.6 g

Fiber: 8.6 g
Carbohydrates: 5.1 g

Protein: 12.9g

34. YOGURT WAFFLES

INGREDIENTS

- 1/2 cup golden flax seeds meal
- 1/2 cup plus 3 tablespoons almond flour
- 1-11/2 tablespoons granulated Erythritol
- 1 tablespoon unsweetened vanilla whey protein powder
- 1/4 teaspoon baking soda
- 1/2 teaspoon organic baking powder
- 1/4 teaspoon xanthan gum
- Salt, as required
- 1 large organic egg, white and yolk separated
- 1 organic whole egg

- 2 tablespoons unsweetened almond milk
- 11/2 tablespoons unsalted butter
- 3 ounces plain Greek yogurt

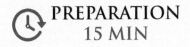 **PREPARATION** 15 MIN

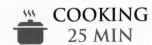 **COOKING** 25 MIN

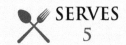 **SERVES** 5

DIRECTIONS

1. Preheat the waffle iron and then grease it.
2. In a large bowl, add the flour, Erythritol, protein powder, baking soda, baking powder, xanthan gum, salt, and mix until well combined.
3. In another bowl or container, put in the egg white and beat until stiff peaks form.
4. In a third bowl, add two egg yolks, whole egg, almond milk, butter, yogurt, and beat until well combined.
5. Place egg mixture into the bowl of the flour mixture and mix until well combined.
6. Gently, fold in the beaten egg whites.
7. Place 1/4 cup of the mixture into preheated waffle iron and cook for about 4–5 minutes or until golden brown.
8. Repeat with the remaining mixture.
9. Serve warm.

Nutritions:

Calories: 265 kcal
Fat: 11.5 g

Fiber: 9.5 g
Carbohydrates: 5.2 g

Protein: 7.5 g

35. GREEN VEGETABLE QUICHE

INGREDIENTS

- 6 organic eggs
- 1/2 cup unsweetened almond milk
- Salt and ground black pepper, as required
- 2 cups fresh baby spinach, chopped
- 1/2 cup green bell pepper, seeded and chopped
- 1 scallion, chopped
- 1/4 cup fresh cilantro, chopped
- 1 tablespoon fresh chives, minced
- 3 tablespoons mozzarella cheese, grated

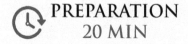 **PREPARATION** 20 MIN   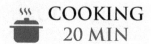 **COOKING** 20 MIN   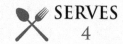 **SERVES** 4

DIRECTIONS

1. Preheat your oven to 400°F.
2. Lightly grease a pie dish.
3. In a bowl, add eggs, almond milk, salt, and black pepper, and beat until well combined. Set aside.
4. In another bowl, add the vegetables and herbs and mix well.
5. At the bottom of the prepared pie dish, place the veggie mixture evenly and top with the egg mixture.
6. Let the quiche bake for about 20 minutes.
7. Remove the pie dish from the oven and immediately sprinkle with the Parmesan cheese.
8. Set aside for about 5 minutes before slicing.
9. Cut into desired sized wedges and serve warm.

Nutritions:

Calories: 298 kcal
Fat: 10.4 g

Fiber: 5.9 g
Carbohydrates: 4.1 g

Protein: 7.9 g

36. CHEESY BROCCOLI MUFFINS

INGREDIENTS

- 2 tablespoons unsalted butter
- 6 large organic eggs
- 1/2 cup heavy whipping cream
- 1/2 cup Parmesan cheese, grated
- Salt and ground black pepper, as required
- 11/4 cups broccoli, chopped
- 2 tablespoons fresh parsley, chopped
- 1/2 cup Swiss cheese, grated

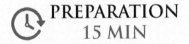 **PREPARATION** 15 MIN

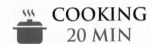 **COOKING** 20 MIN

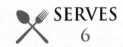 **SERVES** 6

DIRECTIONS

1. Grease a 12-cup muffin tin.
2. In a bowl or container, put in the cream, eggs, Parmesan cheese, salt, and black pepper, and beat until well combined.
3. Divide the broccoli and parsley in the bottom of each prepared muffin cup evenly.
4. Top with the egg mixture, followed by the Swiss cheese.
5. Let the muffins bake for about 20 minutes, rotating the pan once halfway through.
6. Carefully, invert the muffins onto a serving platter and serve warm.

Nutritions:

Calories: 241 kcal
Fat: 11.5 g

Fiber: 8.5 g
Carbohydrates: 4.1 g

Protein: 11.1 g

37. BERRY CHOCOLATE BREAKFAST BOWL

INGREDIENTS

- 1/2 cup strawberries, fresh or frozen
- 1/2 cup blueberries, fresh or frozen
- 1 cup unsweetened almond milk
- Sugar-free maple syrup to taste
- 2 tbsp. unsweetened cocoa powder
- 1 tbsp. cashew nuts for topping

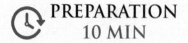 **PREPARATION**
10 MIN

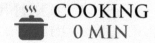 **COOKING**
0 MIN

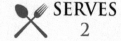 **SERVES**
2

DIRECTIONS

1. The berries must be divided into four bowls, pour on the almond milk.
2. Drizzle with the maple syrup and sprinkle the cocoa powder on top, a tablespoon per bowl.
3. Top with the cashew nuts and enjoy immediately.

Nutritions:

Calories: 287 kcal
Fat: 5.9 g

Fiber: 11.4 g
Carbohydrates: 3.1 g

Protein: 4.2 g

38. "COCO-NUT" GRANOLA

INGREDIENTS

- 2 cups shredded unsweetened coconut
- 1 cup sliced almonds
- 1 cup raw sunflower seeds
- 1/2 cup raw pumpkin seeds
- 1/2 cup walnuts
- 1/2 cup melted coconut oil
- 10 drops liquid stevia
- 1 teaspoon ground cinnamon
- 1/2 teaspoon ground nutmeg

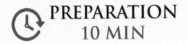 **PREPARATION**
10 MIN

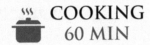 **COOKING**
60 MIN

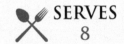 **SERVES**
8

DIRECTIONS

1. Preheat the oven to 250°F. Line 2 baking sheets with parchment paper. Set aside.
2. Toss all the ingredients together.
3. The granola will then be put into baking sheets and spread out evenly.
4. Bake the granola for about 1 hr.

Nutritions:

Calories: 131 kcal
Fat: 4.1 g

Fiber: 5.8 g
Carbohydrates: 2.8 g

Protein: 5.6 g

39. BACON ARTICHOKE OMELET

INGREDIENTS

- 6 eggs, beaten
- 2 tablespoons heavy (whipping) cream
- 8 bacon slices, cooked and chopped
- 1 tablespoon olive oil
- 1/4 cup chopped onion
- 1/2 cup chopped artichoke hearts (canned, packed in water)
- Sea salt
- Freshly ground black pepper

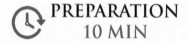 **PREPARATION** 10 MIN

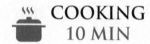 **COOKING** 10 MIN

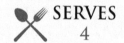 **SERVES** 4

DIRECTIONS

1. In a bowl or container, the eggs, heavy cream, and bacon must be mixed.
2. Heat olive oil then sauté the onion until tender, about 3 minutes.
3. Pour the egg mixture into the skillet for 1 minute.
4. Cook the omelet, lifting the edges with a spatula to let the uncooked egg flow underneath, for 2 minutes.
5. Sprinkle the artichoke hearts on top and flip the omelet.
6. Cook for 4 minutes more until the egg is firm.
7. Flip the omelet over again, so the artichoke hearts are on top.
8. Remove from the heat, cut the omelet into quarters, and season with salt and black pepper.
9. Transfer the omelet to plates and serve.

Nutritions:

Calories: 314 kcal
Fat: 7.1 g

Fiber: 5.4 g
Carbohydrates: 3.1 g

Protein: 8.5 g

40. SPINACH-MUSHROOM FRITTATA

INGREDIENTS

- 2 tablespoons olive oil
- 1 cup sliced fresh mushrooms
- 1 cup shredded spinach
- 6 bacon slices, cooked and chopped
- 10 large eggs, beaten
- 1/2 cup crumbled goat cheese
- Sea salt
- Freshly ground black pepper

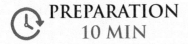 **PREPARATION**
10 MIN

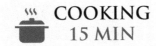 **COOKING**
15 MIN

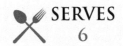 **SERVES**
6

DIRECTIONS

1. Preheat the oven to 350°F.
2. Heat olive oil and sauté the mushrooms until lightly browned about 3 minutes.
3. Add the spinach and bacon and sauté until the greens are wilted about 1 minute.
4. Add the eggs and cook, lifting the edges of the frittata with a spatula so uncooked egg flow underneath, for 3 to 4 minutes.
5. Sprinkle with crumbled goat cheese and season lightly with salt and pepper.
6. Bake until set and lightly browned, about 15 minutes.
7. Remove the frittata from the oven, and let it stand for 5 minutes.
8. Cut into six wedges and serve immediately.

Nutritions:

Calories: 312 kcal
Fat: 6.8 g

Fiber: 5.1 g
Carbohydrates: 3.1 g

Protein: 10.5 g

41. CRÊPES WITH LEMON-BUTTERY SYRUP

INGREDIENTS

- 6 ounces mascarpone cheese, softened
- 6 eggs
- 1 1/2 tbsp. granulated swerve
- 1/4 cup almond flour
- 1 tsp. baking soda
- 1 tsp. baking powder
- For the Syrup
- 3/4 cup water
- 2 tbsp. lemon juice
- 1 tbsp. butter
- 3/4 cup swerve, powdered
- 1 tbsp. vanilla extract
- 1/2 tsp. xanthan gum

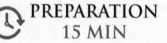 **PREPARATION** 15 MIN

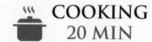 **COOKING** 20 MIN

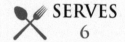 **SERVES** 6

DIRECTIONS

1. With the use of an electric mixer, mix all crepes ingredients until well incorporated.
2. Use melted butter to grease a frying pan and set over medium heat; cook the crepes.
3. Flip over and cook the other side for a further 2 minutes; repeat the remaining batter.
4. Put the crepes on a plate.
5. In the same pan, mix swerve, butter and water; simmer for 6 minutes as you stir.
6. Transfer the mixture to a blender and a 1/4 teaspoon xanthan gum and vanilla extract and mix well.
7. Place in the remaining 1/4 teaspoon xanthan gum and allow sitting until the syrup is thick.

Nutritions:

Calories: 312 kcal
Fat: 11.5 g

Fiber: 3.8 g
Carbohydrates: 2.4 g

Protein: 5.1 g

42. FLAXSEED, MAPLE & PUMPKIN MUFFIN

INGREDIENTS

- 1 tbsp. cinnamon
- 1 cup pure pumpkin puree
- 1 tbsp. pumpkin pie spice
- 2 tbsp. coconut oil
- 1 egg
- 1/2 tbsp. baking powder
- 1/2 tsp. salt
- 1/2 tsp. apple cider vinegar
- 1/2 tsp. vanilla extract
- 1/3 cup erythritol
- 1 1/4 cup flaxseeds (ground)
- 1/4 cup Maple Syrup

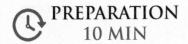 **PREPARATION** 10 MIN

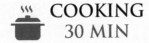 **COOKING** 30 MIN

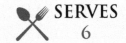 **SERVES** 6

DIRECTIONS

1. Line ten muffin tins with ten muffin liners and preheat oven to 350oF.
2. All the ingredients must be blended until smooth and creamy, around 5 minutes.
3. Evenly divide batter into prepared muffin tins.
4. Pop in the oven and let it bake for 20 minutes or until tops are lightly browned.
5. Let it cool. Evenly divide into suggested servings and place in meal prep containers.

Nutritions:

Calories: 241 kcal
Fat: 11.3 g

Fiber: 15.9 g
Carbohydrates: 3.1 g

Protein: 8.9g

43. ONION CHEESE MUFFINS

INGREDIENTS

- 1/4 cup Colby jack cheese, shredded
- 1/4 cup shallots, minced
- 1/2 tsp. salt
- 1 cup almond flour
- 1 egg
- 3 tbsp. melted butter
- 3 tbsp. sour cream

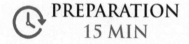 **PREPARATION**
15 MIN

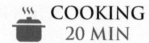 **COOKING**
20 MIN

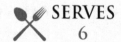 **SERVES**
6

DIRECTIONS

1. Line 6 muffin tins with six muffin liners. Set aside and preheat oven to 350oF.
2. In a bowl, stir the dry and wet ingredients alternately. Mix well.
3. Scoop a spoonful of the batter to the prepared muffin tins.
4. Bake for 20 minutes in the oven until golden brown.

Nutritions:

Calories: 241 kcal
Fat: 5.1 g

Fiber: 2.6 g
Carbohydrates: 3.1 g

Protein: 4.2 g

44. CAJUN CRABMEAT FRITTATA

INGREDIENTS

- 1 tbsp. olive oil
- 1 onion, chopped
- 4 ounces crabmeat, chopped
- 1 tsp. Cajun seasoning
- 6 large eggs, slightly beaten
- 1/2 cup Greek yogurt

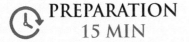 **PREPARATION**
15 MIN

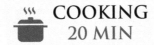 **COOKING**
20 MIN

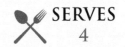 **SERVES**
4

DIRECTIONS

1. Let the oven preheat to 350°F/175°C, then set a large skillet over medium heat and warm the oil.
2. Add in onion and sauté until soft; place in crabmeat and cook for two more minutes.
3. Season with Cajun seasoning.
4. Evenly distribute the ingredients at the bottom of the skillet.
5. Whisk the eggs with yogurt.
6. Transfer to the skillet.
7. Put it in the oven and let the frittata bake for about 18 minutes or until eggs are cooked.
8. Slice into wedges and serve warm.

Nutritions:

Calories: 256 kcal
Fat: 4.9 g

Fiber: 2.9 g
Carbohydrates: 3.1 g

Protein: 8.9 g

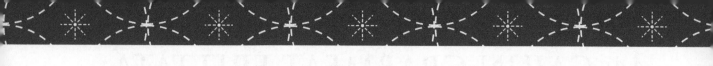

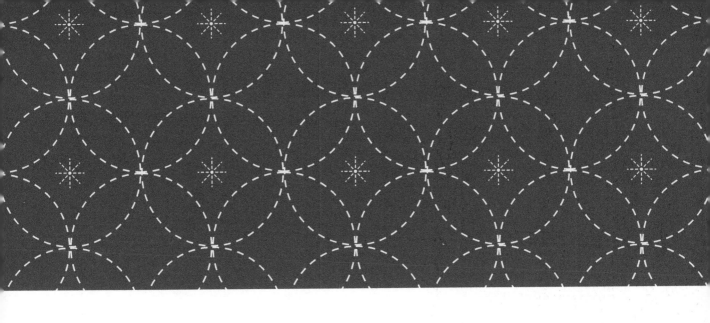

CHAPTER 7
LUNCH

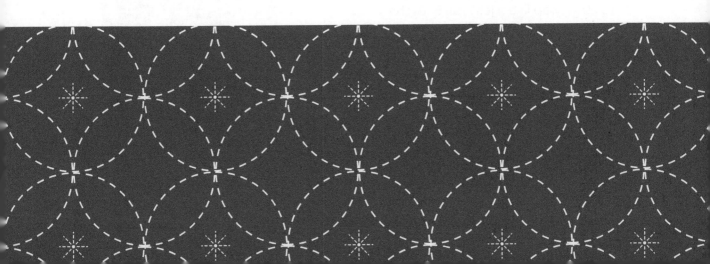

45. KETO CHICKEN CLUB LETTUCE WRAP

INGREDIENTS

- 1 head iceberg lettuce with the core and outer leaves removed
- 1 tbsp. mayonnaise
- 6 slices of organic chicken or turkey breast
- Bacon (2 cooked strips, halved)
- Tomato (just 2 slices)

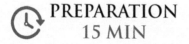 **PREPARATION** 15 MIN

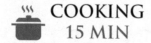 **COOKING** 15 MIN

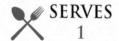 **SERVES** 1

DIRECTIONS

1. Line your working surface with a large slice of parchment paper.
2. Layer 6-8 large leaves of lettuce in the center of the paper to make a base of around 9-10 inches.
3. Spread the mayo in the center and lay with chicken or turkey, bacon, and tomato.
4. Starting with the end closest to you, roll the wrap like a jelly roll with the parchment paper as your guide. Keep it tight and halfway through, roll tuck in the ends of the wrap.
5. When it is completely wrapped, roll the rest of the parchment paper around it, and use a knife to cut it in half.

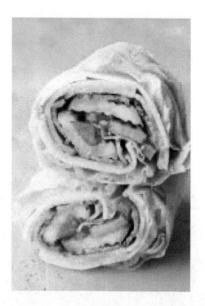

Nutritions:

Net carbs: 4 g
Fiber: 2 g

Fat: 78 g
Protein: 28 g

Calories: 837 kcal

46. KETO BROCCOLI SALAD

INGREDIENTS

For your salad:
- Broccoli (2 medium-sized heads, florets chunked)
- Red Cabbage (2 cups shredded well)
- Sliced Almonds (0.5 cups, roasted)
- Green Onions (1 stalk, sliced)
- Raisins (0.5 cups)

For your orange almond dressing:
- Orange Juice (0.33 cup)
- Almond Butter (0.25 cup)
- Coconut Aminos (2 tablespoons)
- Shallot (1; small-sized, chopped finely)
- Salt (a half-teaspoon)

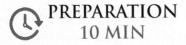 **PREPARATION**
10 MIN

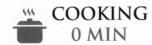 **COOKING**
0 MIN

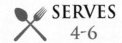 **SERVES**
4-6

DIRECTIONS

1. Use a food processor to pulse together salt, shallot, amino, nut butter, and OJ. Make sure it is perfectly smooth.
2. Use a medium-sized bowl to combine other ingredients. Toss it with dressing and serve.

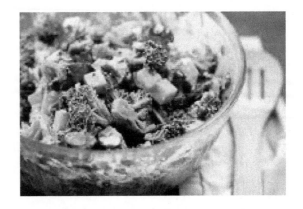

Nutritions:

Net carbs: 13 g
Fiber: 0 g

Fat: 94 g
Protein: 22 g

Calories: 1022 kcal

47. KETO SHEET PAN CHICKEN AND RAINBOW VEGGIES

INGREDIENTS

- Nonstick spray
- Chicken Breasts (1 pound, boneless & skinless)
- Sesame Oil (1 tablespoon)
- Soy Sauce (2 tablespoons)
- Honey (2 tablespoons)
- Red Pepper (2; medium-sized, sliced)
- Yellow Pepper (2; medium-sized, sliced)
- Carrots (3; medium-sized, sliced)
- Broccoli (half-a-head cut up)
- 2 Red Onions (medium-size and sliced)
- EVOO (2 tablespoons)
- Pepper & salt (to taste)
- Parsley (0.25 cup, fresh herb, chopped)

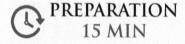 **PREPARATION** 15 MIN

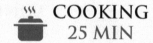 **COOKING** 25 MIN

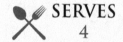 **SERVES** 4

DIRECTIONS

1. Spray cooking spray on a baking sheet and bring the oven to a temperature of 400-degrees
2. Put the chicken in the middle of the sheet. Separately, combine the oil and the soy sauce. Brush the mix over the chicken.
3. As the image above shows, separate your veggies across the plate. Sprinkle with oil and then toss them gently to ensure they are coated. Finally, spice up with pepper & salt.
4. Set tray into the oven and cook for around 25 minutes until all is tender and done throughout.
5. After taking it out of the oven, garnish using parsley. Divide everything between those prep containers paired with your favorite greens.

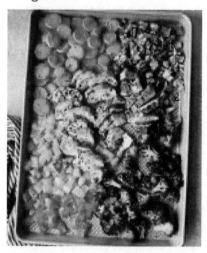

Nutritions:

Net carbs: 9 g

Fiber: 0 g

Fat: 30 g

Protein: 30 g

Calories: 437 kcal

48. SAUSAGE WITH ZUCCHINI NOODLES

INGREDIENTS

- One large zucchini, spiralized into noodles
- 3 oz sausage
- ½ tsp garlic powder
- 4 oz marinara sauce
- 2 tsp grated parmesan cheese

Seasoning:
- 1/3 tsp salt
- 1/8 tsp dried basil
- ¼ tsp Italian seasoning
- 1 tbsp avocado oil

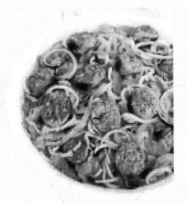

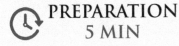 **PREPARATION** 5 MIN

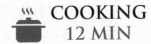 **COOKING** 12 MIN

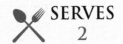 **SERVES** 2

DIRECTIONS

1. Take a skillet pan, place it over medium heat and hot, add sausage, crumble it and cook for 5 minutes until nicely browned.
2. When done, transfer sausage to a bowl, drain the grease, add oil and when hot, add zucchini noodles, sprinkle with garlic, toss until mixed, and cook for 3 minutes zucchini begins to tender.
3. Add marinara sauce, return sausage into the pan, toss until mixed, add salt, basil, and Italian seasoning, stir until mixed and cook for 2 to 3 minutes until hot.
4. When done, distribute marinara noodles between two plates, sprinkle with cheese, and then serve.

Nutritions:

Carbohydrates: 0.4 g
Protein: 5.6 g

Fats: 4.9 g
Calories: 69 kcal

49. KETO CRISPY ROSEMARY CHICKEN DRUMSTICKS

INGREDIENTS

- 12 chicken drumsticks
- 4 tbsp. olive oil
- 4 tbsp. rosemary leaves
- 2 tsp. salt

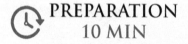 **PREPARATION**
10 MIN

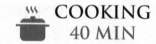 **COOKING**
40 MIN

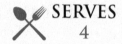 **SERVES**
4

DIRECTIONS

1. Preheat oven to 450 F.
2. Rub salt and rosemary on each chicken drumstick the blend and spot on a lubed heating plate.
3. Make sure the drumsticks are not contacting each other on the plate. Drizzle the olive oil or avocado oil over the chicken drumsticks.
4. Prepare for 40 minutes until the skin is firm.

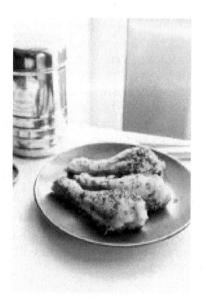

Nutritions:

Calories: 473 kcal
Fat: 32 g

Carbs: 6 g
Protein: 42 g

50. BAKED PESTO CHICKEN

INGREDIENTS

- Four chicken breasts (about 1½ lb.)
- 3 tbsp. basil pesto
- 8 oz. mozzarella
- ½ tsp. salt
- ¼ tsp. black pepper

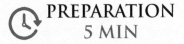
PREPARATION
5 MIN

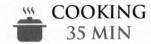
COOKING
35 MIN

SERVES
4

DIRECTIONS

1. Preheat oven to 350 F.
2. Coat heating dish with cooking spray. Put the chicken in the base in a single layer and sprinkle with the salt and pepper.
3. Spread the pesto on the bird. Put the mozzarella on top.
4. Heat for 35-45 minutes until the cheddar is bubbly.
5. Serve.

Nutritions:

Calories: 471 kcal
Fat: 22 g

Carbs: 3.4 g
Protein: 61 g

51. CHEESEBURGER SKILLET WITH BACON & MUSHROOMS

INGREDIENTS

- Two slices Canadian bacon, chopped
- 1/2 cup shallots, sliced
- 1 garlic clove, minced
- 1-pound ground pork
- Sea salt and ground black pepper
- 1/3 cup vegetable broth
- 1/4 cup white wine
- 6 ounces Cremini mushrooms, sliced
- 1/2 cup cream cheese

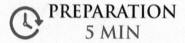 **PREPARATION** 5 MIN

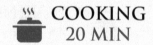 **COOKING** 20 MIN

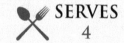 **SERVES** 4

DIRECTIONS

1. Heat a cast-iron skillet.
2. Cook the bacon and reserve the bacon and tablespoon of fat. Then, sauté the shallots and garlic in 1 tablespoon of bacon fat until tender and fragrant.
3. Add the ground pork, salt, and black pepper to the skillet. Cook for 4 to 5 minutes or until ground meat is nicely browned.
4. Add broth, wine, and mushrooms. Close the lid, then cook for 8 to 9 minutes over medium flame.
5. Turn off the heat. Add cream cheese and stir to combine. Serve topped with the reserved bacon. Enjoy!

Nutritions:

Calories: 463 kcal
Fat: 60 g

Carbs: 4.7 g
Fiber: 0.8 g

Protein: 36.2 g

52. CHICKEN COBB SALAD

INGREDIENTS

- 1/2 lb. Chicken, sliced
- ¼ tsp. Smoked Paprika
- 2 Eggs, hardboiled & chopped
- 2 tbsp. Olive Oil
- Salt & Pepper, as needed
- 4 Ham slices
- ¼ tsp. Onion Powder
- ½ of 1 Avocado, medium & sliced
- ½ cup Cucumbers, chopped
- 3 cups Greens of your choice
- ½ cup Cherry Tomatoes quartered

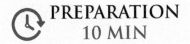 **PREPARATION 10 MIN**   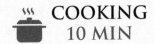 **COOKING 10 MIN**   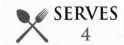 **SERVES 4**

DIRECTIONS

1. First, marinate the chicken with salt, onion powder, pepper, and smoked paprika. Set it aside.
2. Heat a large cast-iron skillet over medium-low heat.
3. Stir in the chicken and sear it for 4 minutes on each side or until the chicken is cooked. Slice it once cooled.
4. Place all the remaining ingredients needed to make the salad along with the chicken.
5. Serve it with the dressing just before serving.
6. Enjoy.

Nutritions:

Calories: 130 Kcal   Fiber: 4 g   Sugar: 4 g
Proteins: 5 g   Fat: 7 g   Sodium: 454 mg

53. KETO BAKED SALMON WITH LEMON AND BUTTER

INGREDIENTS

- 1 pound salmon
- 1 lemon
- 3 oz. Butter
- 1 tablespoon olive oil
- Ground black pepper and sea salt

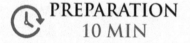
PREPARATION
10 MIN

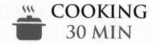
COOKING
30 MIN

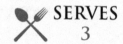
SERVES
3

DIRECTIONS

1. Grease a large-sized baking dish with the olive oil and preheat your oven to 400°f.
2. Place the salmon on the baking dish, preferably skin-side down. Generously season with pepper and salt to taste.
3. Thinly slice the lemon and place the slices over the salmon. Cover the fish with ½ of the butter, preferably in very thin slices.
4. Bake until it is opaque, for 25 to 30 minutes, on the middle rack.
5. Now, over moderate heat in a small saucepan; heat the remaining butter until it begins to bubble. Immediately remove the pan from heat; set aside and let cool a bit. Gently add in some of the freshly squeezed lemon juice.
6. Serve the cooked fish with some of the prepared lemon butter and enjoy.

Nutritions:

Calories: 576 kcal
Total Fat: 46 g
Saturated Fat: 22 g

Total Carbohydrates: 1.3 g
Dietary Fiber: 0.4 g
Sugars: 0.4 g

Protein: 31 g

54. KETOGENIC SPICY OYSTER

INGREDIENTS

- 12 oysters shucked
- 1 tablespoon olive oil
- 7-8 basil leaves, fresh
- 1 tablespoon garlic chili paste
- 1/8 teaspoon salt

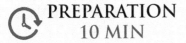 **PREPARATION**
10 MIN

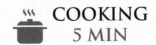 **COOKING**
5 MIN

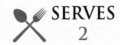 **SERVES**
2

DIRECTIONS

1. Combine olive oil with garlic chili paste and salt in a medium-size mixing bowl; mix well.
2. Add oysters into the prepared sauce; turning them several times until thoroughly coated.
3. Create a bed for the oysters to cook by spreading the basil leaves out on an oven-safe dish.
4. Transfer the oysters and sauce over the bed of basil leaves; spreading them in a single layer on the dish.
5. Turn on the broiler over high heat.
6. Place the dish on the top rack (approximately a few inches away from the broiler) and broil for a few minutes.
7. Once done; immediately remove them from the oven. Serve hot and enjoy.

Nutritions:

Calories: 102 kcal
Total Fat: 8 g
Saturated Fat: 2.5 g

Total Carbohydrates: 2 g
Dietary Fiber: 0 g
Sugars: 0.3 g

Protein: 4 g

55. GARLIC LIME MAHI-MAHI

INGREDIENTS

- 4 mahi-mahi filets (approximately 1 to 1 ¼ pounds)
- Zest and juice of 1 large lime, fresh
- ¼ cup avocado oil
- 3 cloves garlic, minced
- 1/8 teaspoon each of ground black pepper and fine grain sea salt

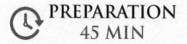 **PREPARATION**
45 MIN

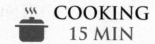 **COOKING**
15 MIN

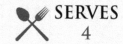 **SERVES**
4

DIRECTIONS

1. For the marinade: thoroughly combine the entire ingredients (except the filets) together in a small-sized mixing bowl. Pour the mixture on top of filets in a large zip-lock bag or large shallow dish. Marinate for 30 minutes, at room temperature.
2. Pour the marinade into a large sauté pan (preferably with a cover) and heat it over medium heat. Once hot; carefully add the filets into the hot pan; cover and cook the filets for a couple of minutes, until cooked through.
3. Immediately remove the sauté pan from heat; set aside and let rest for 5 minutes, covered. Serve warm and enjoy.

Nutritions:

Calories: 248
Total Fat: 14 g
Saturated Fat: 1.7 g

Total Carbohydrates: 0.7 g   Protein: 24 g
Dietary Fiber: 0.1 g
Sugars: 0 g

56. FISH AND LEEK SAUTÉ

INGREDIENTS

- 1 leek, chopped
- 2 trout fillets, diced (approximately 8 oz.)
- 1 tablespoon tamari soy sauce
- 1 teaspoon ginger, grated
- 1 tablespoon avocado oil
- Salt to taste

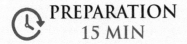 **PREPARATION 15 MIN**   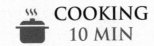 **COOKING 10 MIN**   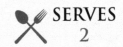 **SERVES 2**

DIRECTIONS

1. Over moderate heat in a large skillet; heat the avocado oil until hot. Once done; add and sauté the chopped leek for a few minutes, until turn soften.
2. Immediately add the diced trout with grated ginger, tamari sauce and salt to taste.
3. Continue to sauté the trout until it's not translucent anymore and cooked through.
4. Serve immediately and enjoy.

Nutritions:

Calories: 175 kcal
Total Fat: 7.6 g
Saturated Fat: 1.5 g

Total Carbohydrates: 5.2 g
Dietary Fiber: 0.8 g
Sugars: 1.7 g

Protein: 21 g

57. SMOKED SALMON SALAD

INGREDIENTS

- 2 oz. Smoked salmon
- 1 lemon slice
- 4 olives
- 1 teaspoon pink peppercorns, crushed lightly
- A handful of arugula salad leaves, fresh

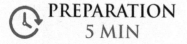 **PREPARATION**
5 MIN

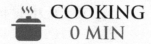 **COOKING**
0 MIN

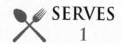 **SERVES**
1

DIRECTIONS

1. Place the olives and salad leaves into a large plate or shallow bowl.
2. Arrange the smoked salmon over the salad.
3. Sprinkle the top of smoked salmon with lightly crushed pink peppercorns.
4. Garnish your salad with a lemon slice; serve immediately and enjoy.

Nutritions:

Calories: 149 kcal
Total Fat: 5.2 g
Saturated Fat: 1.4 g

Total Carbohydrates: 4 g
Dietary Fiber: 1.7 g
Sugars: 3.4 g

Protein: 11 g

58. KETO BAKED SALMON WITH PESTO

INGREDIENTS

- 1 oz. Green pesto
- ½ pound salmon
- Pepper and salt to taste

For Green Sauce:
- ¼ cup Greek yogurt
- 1 oz. green pesto
- ¼ teaspoon garlic
- Pepper and salt to taste

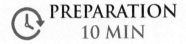 **PREPARATION**
10 MIN

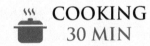 **COOKING**
30 MIN

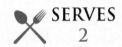 **SERVES**
2

DIRECTIONS

1. Preheat your oven to 400°f.
2. Arrange the salmon in a well-greased baking dish, preferably skin-side down. Spread the pesto over the salmon and then, sprinkle with pepper and salt to taste.
3. Bake in the preheated oven until the salmon flakes easily with a fork, for 25 to 30 minutes.
4. In the meantime, stir the entire sauce ingredients together in a large bowl. Serve the cooked fish with some of the prepared sauce and enjoy.

Nutritions:

Calories: 274 kcal
Total Fat: 21 g
Saturated Fat: 3.9 g

Total Carbohydrates: 2.9 g
Dietary Fiber: 0.6 g
Sugars: 1.7 g

Protein: 26 g

59. ROASTED SALMON WITH PARMESAN DILL CRUST

INGREDIENTS

- ½ pound salmon; cut into pieces
- 1 tablespoon dill weed
- ¼ cup cottage cheese
- 1 tablespoon olive oil
- ¼ cup parmesan cheese, grated

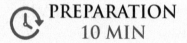 **PREPARATION** 10 MIN   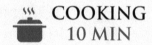 **COOKING** 10 MIN    **SERVES** 2

DIRECTIONS

1. Preheat your oven to 450°f.
2. Combine cottage cheese with parmesan cheese, olive oil and dill in a large-sized mixing bowl; mix well.
3. Using a baking sheet lined with aluminum foil, arrange the salmon pieces on it.
4. Smear ½ of the cottage cheese mixture over the salmon.
5. Roast in the preheated oven until the fish flakes easily and the crust is brown, for 10 minutes.
6. Serve the cooked fish with the remaining prepared sauce and enjoy.

Nutritions:

Calories: 352 kcal
Total Fat: 22 g
Saturated Fat: 6.6 g

Total Carbohydrates: 5.7 g
Dietary Fiber: 1.5 g
Sugars: 0.5 g

Protein: 33 g

60. ARTICHOKE DIP

INGREDIENTS

- Frozen spinach – 10-ounce
- Artichoke hearts, chopped – 14 ounces
- Cloves of garlic, peeled – 3
- Onion powder – 1 teaspoon
- Mayonnaise, full-fat – ½ cup
- Parmesan cheese, grated and full-fat – 12 ounces
- Cream cheese, full-fat – 8 ounces
- Sour cream, full-fat – ½ cup
- Swiss cheese, grated, full-fat – 12 ounces
- Chicken broth, organic – ½ cup

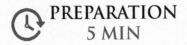 **PREPARATION** 5 MIN   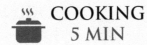 **COOKING** 5 MIN   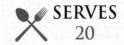 **SERVES** 20

DIRECTIONS

1. Switch on an instant pot, place all the ingredients except for Swiss cheese and parmesan cheese and stir until just mixed.
2. Shut an instant pot with its lid, sealed completely, press the manual button and cook eggs for 4 minutes at high pressure.
3. When finished, let the pressure release for 5 minutes, then do a quick pressure release and open the instant pot.
4. Add swiss and parmesan cheese into the instant pot and stir well until cheeses melt and are well combined.
5. Serve immediately.

Nutritions:

Calories: 230.7 kcal
Fat: 18.7 g
Protein: 12.6 g

Net carbs: 2.6 g
Fiber: 0.7 g

61. TACO MEAT

INGREDIENTS

- Ground turkey – 2-pound
- Diced white onion – 1/2 cup
- Diced red bell pepper – 1/2 cup
- Tomato sauce, unsalted – 1 cup
- Taco seasoning – 1 1/2 tablespoon
- Fajita seasoning – 1 ½ tablespoon
- Avocado oil – 1 teaspoon

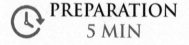 **PREPARATION**
5 MIN

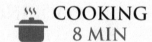 **COOKING**
8 MIN

 **SERVES**
8

DIRECTIONS

1. Switch on the instant pot, grease pot with oil, press the 'sauté/simmer' button, wait until the oil is hot and add the ground turkey and cook for 7 to 10 minutes or until nicely browned.
2. Then add remaining ingredients, stir until mixed and press the 'keep warm' button.
3. Shut the instant pot with its lid in the sealed position, then press the 'manual' button, press '+/-' to set the cooking time to 8 minutes and cook at a high-pressure setting; when the pressure builds in the pot, the cooking timer will start.
4. When the instant pot buzzes, press the 'keep warm' button, do a quick pressure release and open the lid.
5. Transfer taco meat to a bowl, top with avocado slices, garnish with cilantro and serve.

Nutritions:

Calories: 231 kcal
Fat: 14 g
Protein: 21 g

Net carbs: 2.5 g
Fiber: 1.5 g

62. GREEN BEANS WITH BACON

INGREDIENTS

- 5 slices bacon, chopped
- 6 cups Green beans, halved
- 1 teaspoon salt
- 1 teaspoon ground black pepper
- 1/4 cup water
- 2 tablespoons avocado oil

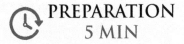 **PREPARATION** 5 MIN   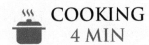 **COOKING** 4 MIN   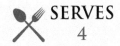 **SERVES** 4

DIRECTIONS

1. Switch on the instant pot, place all the ingredients in it except for oil and stir until mixed.
2. Shut the instant pot with its lid in the sealed position, then press the 'manual' button, press '+/-' to set the cooking time to 4 minutes and cook at a high-pressure setting; when the pressure builds in the pot, the cooking timer will start.
3. When the instant pot buzzes, press the 'keep warm' button, do a quick pressure release and open the lid.
4. Transfer the greens and bacon to a dish, drizzle with oil, toss until well coated and serve.

Nutritions:

Calories: 153 kcal
Fat: 9.2 g
Protein: 7 g

Net carbs: 4.4 g
Fiber: 5.6 g

63. MEATBALLS

INGREDIENTS

- Ground beef, pastured – 1 1/4 pounds
- Medium white onion, peeled, minced – 1/2
- Minced garlic – 1 tablespoon
- Ground black pepper – 1/2 teaspoon
- Salt – 1 teaspoon
- Crushed red pepper flakes – 1 teaspoon
- Fresh rosemary, chopped – 1/4 cup
- Butter, grass-fed, unsalted, softened – 2 tablespoons
- Apple cider vinegar – 1 tablespoon

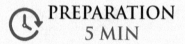 **PREPARATION**
5 MIN

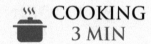 **COOKING**
3 MIN

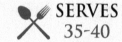 **SERVES**
35-40

DIRECTIONS

1. Set oven to 350 degrees f and let preheat until meatballs are ready to bake.
2. Place all the ingredients in a bowl, stir until well combined, then shape the mixture into meatballs, 1 tablespoon per meatball, and place them on a baking tray lined with parchment sheet.
3. Place the baking tray into the oven and bake the meatballs for 20 minutes or until thoroughly cooked and nicely golden brown.
4. When done, cool the meatballs, then place them in batches in the meal prepare glass containers and refrigerate for up to 5 days or freeze for 3 months.
5. Reheat the meatballs in the oven at 400 degrees f for 7 to 10 minutes or until hot.
6. Serve meatballs with zucchini noodles.

Nutritions:

Calories: 474 kcal
Fat: 21.7 g
Protein: 61.3 g

Net carbs: 3.1 g
Fiber: 2.5 g

64. KETO CHEESESTEAK CASSEROLE

INGREDIENTS

- 4 oz. Butter
- 10 oz. Mushrooms
- 1 yellow onion
- 2 green bell peppers
- 1 pound ribeye steak, thinly sliced
- 1 glove garlic
- 1 tbsp. Italian seasoning
- 1 tsp. Chili flakes
- 7 oz. Shredded provolone cheese
- Salt and pepper
- 4 tbsp. Unsweetened marinara sauce
- 1/2 teaspoon olive oil for drizzle
- Green leafies for topping

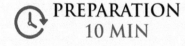 **PREPARATION** 10 MIN

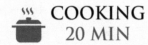 **COOKING** 20 MIN

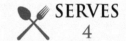 **SERVES** 4

DIRECTIONS

1. Preheat oven to 450°f.
2. Slice or chop mushrooms. Finely chop onion and bell pepper.
3. Fry the vegetables in butter until slightly soft. Put aside.
4. Slice the meat and fry in the same frying pan. Add the garlic and spices. Season with salt and pepper.
5. Return the veggies to the pan and stir.
6. Place everything in a greased baking dish and sprinkle the cheese on top.
7. Bake for 15 – 20 minutes or until the casserole turns golden brown.
8. Drizzle marinara sauce on top and serve with leafy greens and olive oil.

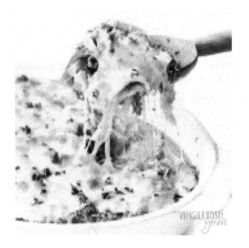

Nutritions:

Calories: 806 kcal
Fat: 68 g
Protein: 40 g

Carb: 9 g

65. BALSAMIC ROAST BEEF

INGREDIENTS

- 1 ¾ pound boneless round roast
- 1 cup beef broth
- 1 tbsp. Stevia
- 1 tbsp. Soy sauce
- 1 tbsp. Worcestershire sauce
- 4 cloves garlic, chopped
- 1/4 tsp. Red pepper flakes

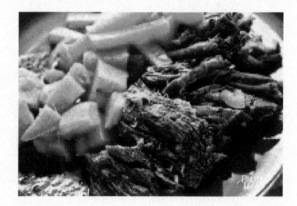

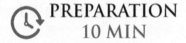 **PREPARATION**
10 MIN

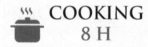 **COOKING**
8 H

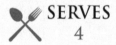 **SERVES**
4

DIRECTIONS

1. Place the roast beef in the slow cooker.
2. In a mixing bowl, mix all other ingredients and pour over the roast.
3. Let it sit in the slow cooker for six to eight hours.
4. Once cooked, remove from the slow cooker and break the meat apart.
5. You can add a dollop of sour cream and chopped scallions to top off each serving.

Nutritions:

Calories: 355 kcal
Protein: 59 g
Fat: 9.7 g

Carbohydrates: 8 g

66. GREEK STYLE LAMB CHOPS

INGREDIENTS

- 1 tbsp. Black pepper
- 1 tbsp. Dried oregano
- 1 tbsp. Minced garlic
- 2 tbsp. Lemon juice
- 2 tsp. Olive oil
- 2 tsp. Seal salt
- 8 pieces of lamb loin chops, around 4 ounces

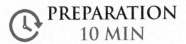 **PREPARATION**
10 MIN

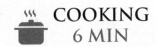 **COOKING**
6 MIN

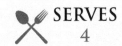 **SERVES**
4

DIRECTIONS

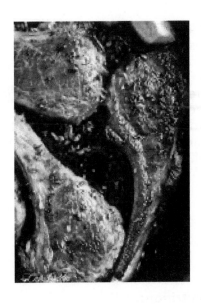

1. In a big bowl or dish, combine the black pepper, salt, minced garlic, lemon juice and oregano. Then rub it equally on all sides of the lamb chops.
2. Then place a skillet on high heat. After a minute, coat the skillet with the cooking spray and place the lamb chops in the skillet. Sear chops for a minute on each side.
3. Lower heat to medium; continue cooking chops for 2 -3 minutes per side until the desired doneness is reached.
4. Let the chops rest for five minutes before serving.

Nutritions:

Calories: 457 kcal   Carbs: 4 g
Protein: 63 g
Fat: 9 g

67. ASIAN BEEF SHORT RIBS

INGREDIENTS

- 2 pounds beef short ribs
- 1 cup water
- 1 onion, sliced
- 1 tbsp. Szechuan peppercorns
- 2 tbsp. Curry powder   3 tbsp. Coconut amino
- 6 pieces star anise
- 6 tbsp. Sesame oil
- Salt and pepper to taste

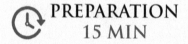 **PREPARATION** 15 MIN

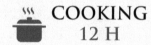 **COOKING** 12 H

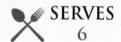 **SERVES** 6

DIRECTIONS

1. Place all ingredients except for the sesame oil in the instant pot.
2. Close the lid and make sure that the steam release valve is set to "venting".
3. Press the "slow cook" button and adjust the cooking time to 12 hours.
4. Once cooked, remove from pot and place into serving dishes. Drizzle with sesame oil, serve.

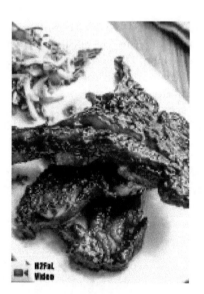

Nutritions:

Calories: 592 kcal   Carbs: 6 g
Protein: 47 g
Fat: 44 g

68. BUFFALO TURKEY BALLS

INGREDIENTS

- 2 eggs
- 1 pound ground turkey
- 1/2 cup hot sauce
- 1/2 stick unsalted butter
- 1/4 cup almond flour
- 3 tbsp. Blue cheese, crumbled
- 2 oz. Whipped cream cheese

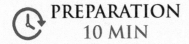 **PREPARATION 10 MIN**   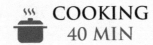 **COOKING 40 MIN**   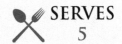 **SERVES 5**

DIRECTIONS

1. Preheat oven to 350°f.
2. Mix the turkey meat, cream cheese, egg, blue cheese and almond flour in a mixing bowl. Mix well and evenly divide into 20 small meatballs.
3. Place the meatballs on a greased baking pan.
4. Bake for 15 minutes.
5. While the meatballs are cooking, make the sauce by mixing the butter and hot sauce in a small saucepan.
6. Remove the meatballs from the oven and dip them in the hot sauce.
7. Place the meatballs in the oven and re-bake for another 15 minutes.
8. Remove the meatballs from the oven and place them into serving dishes. Garnish with chopped scallions or parsley.

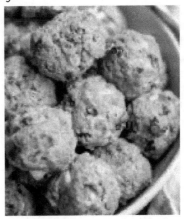

Nutritions:

Calories: 300 kcal
Protein: 30 g
Fat: 18 g

Carbs: 2 g

69. COCONUT CHICKEN

INGREDIENTS

- 2 tablespoons olive oil
- 4 (4 oz.) Chicken breasts, cut into 2-inch chunks
- 1/2 cup chopped sweet onion
- 1 cup coconut milk
- 1 tablespoon curry powder
- 1 teaspoon ground cumin
- 1 teaspoon ground coriander
- 1/4 cup chopped fresh cilantro

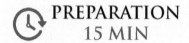 **PREPARATION** 15 MIN   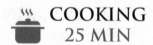 **COOKING** 25 MIN   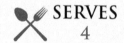 **SERVES** 4

DIRECTIONS

1. Place a large saucepan over medium-high heat and add the olive oil.
2. Sauté the chicken until almost cooked through, about 10 minutes.
3. Add the onion and sauté for an additional 3 minutes.
4. In a medium bowl, whisk together the coconut milk; curry powder cumin, and coriander.
5. Pour the sauce into the saucepan with the chicken and bring the liquid to a boil.
6. Reduce the heat and simmer until the chicken is tender and the sauce has thickened about 10 minutes.
7. Serve the chicken with the sauce, topped with cilantro.

Nutritions:

Calories: 382 kcal   Carbs: 5 g
Fat: 31 g
Protein: 23 g

70. BUFFALO DRUMSTICKS WITH CHILI AIOLI

INGREDIENTS

- 2 lbs. Chicken drumsticks or chicken wings
- 2 tbsp. Olive oil or coconut oil
- 2 tbsp. White wine vinegar
- 1 tbsp. Tomato paste   1 tbsp. Salt
- 1 tsp. Paprika powder
- 1 tbsp. Tabasco
- Butter or olive oil for greasing the baking dish
- Chili aioli
- 2/3 cup mayonnaise
- 1 tbsp. Smoked paprika powder or

smoked chili powder
- 1 garlic clove, minced

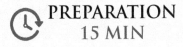 **PREPARATION**
15 MIN

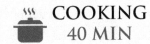 **COOKING**
40 MIN

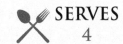 **SERVES**
4

DIRECTIONS

1. Preheat oven to 450°f.
2. Put the drumsticks in a plastic bag.
3. Mix the ingredients for the marinade in a small bowl and pour into the plastic bag. Shake the bag thoroughly and let marinate for 10 minutes at room temperature.
4. Coat a baking dish with oil. Place the drumsticks in the baking dish and let bake for 30-40 minutes or until they are done and have turned a nice color.
5. Mix together mayonnaise, garlic and chili.
6. Serve warm

Nutritions:

Calories: 330 kcal   *Carbs: 2 g*
Fat: 56 g
Protein: 42 g

71. CUCUMBER AVOCADO SALAD WITH BACON

INGREDIENTS

- 2 cups fresh baby spinach, chopped
- 1/2 English cucumber, sliced thin
- 1 small avocado, pitted and chopped
- 1 1/2 tablespoon olive oil
- 1 1/2 tablespoon lemon juice
- Salt and pepper
- 2 slices cooked bacon, chopped

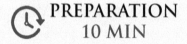 **PREPARATION**
10 MIN

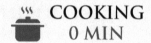 **COOKING**
0 MIN

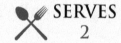 **SERVES**
2

DIRECTIONS

1. Combine the spinach, cucumber, and avocado in a salad bowl. Toss with olive oil, lemon juice, salt and pepper. Top with chopped bacon to serve.

Nutritions:

Calories: 365 kcal
Fat: 24.5 g
Protein: 7 g

Carbs: 13 g
Fiber: 8 g

72. BACON CHEESEBURGER SOUP

INGREDIENTS

- 4 slices uncooked bacon
- 8 ounces ground beef (80% lean)
- 1 medium yellow onion, chopped
- 1 clove garlic, minced
- 3 cups beef broth
- 2 tablespoons tomato paste
- 2 teaspoons dijon mustard
- Salt and pepper
- 1 cup shredded lettuce
- 1/2 cup shredded cheddar cheese

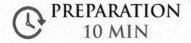 **PREPARATION** 10 MIN

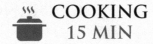 **COOKING** 15 MIN

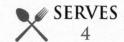 **SERVES** 4

DIRECTIONS

1. Cook the bacon in a saucepan until crisp then drain on paper towels and chop.
2. Reheat the bacon fat in the saucepan and add the beef.
3. Cook until the beef is browned then drains away half the fat.
4. Reheat the saucepan and add the onion and garlic – cook for 6 minutes.
5. Stir in the broth, tomato paste, and mustard then season with salt and pepper.
6. Add the beef and simmer on medium-low for 15 minutes, covered.
7. Spoon into bowls and top with shredded lettuce, cheddar cheese and bacon.

Nutritions:

Calories: 315 kcal
Fat: 20 g
Protein: 27 g

Carbs: 6 g
Fiber: 1 g

73. EGG SALAD OVER LETTUCE

INGREDIENTS

- 3 large hardboiled eggs, cooled
- 1 small stalk celery, diced
- 3 tablespoons mayonnaise
- 1 tablespoon fresh chopped parsley
- 1 teaspoon fresh lemon juice
- Salt and pepper
- 4 cups fresh chopped lettuce

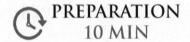 **PREPARATION**
10 MIN

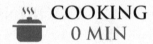 **COOKING**
0 MIN

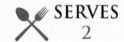 **SERVES**
2

DIRECTIONS

1. Peel and dice the eggs into a mixing bowl.
2. Stir in the celery, mayonnaise, parsley, lemon juice, salt and pepper.
3. Serve spooned over fresh chopped lettuce.

Nutritions:

Calories: 260 kcal
Fat: 23 g
Protein: 10 g

Carbs: 4 g
Fiber: 1 g

74. EGG DROP SOUP

INGREDIENTS

- 5 cups chicken broth
- 4 chicken bouillon cubes
- 1 1/2 tablespoons chili garlic paste
- 6 large eggs, whisked
- 1/2 green onion, sliced

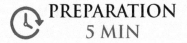 **PREPARATION**
5 MIN

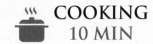 **COOKING**
10 MIN

 **SERVES**
4

DIRECTIONS

1. Crush the bouillon cubes and stir into the broth in a saucepan.
2. Bring it to a boil, and then stir in the chili garlic paste.
3. Cook until steaming, and then remove from heat.
4. While whisking, drizzle in the beaten eggs.
5. Let sit for 2 minutes then serve with sliced green onion.

Nutritions:

Calories: 165 kcal
Fat: 9.5 g
Protein: 16 g

Carbs: 2.5 g
Fiber: 0.5 g

75. SPINACH CAULIFLOWER SOUP

INGREDIENTS

- 1 tablespoon coconut oil
- 1 small yellow onion, chopped
- 2 cloves garlic, minced
- 2 cups chopped cauliflower
- 8 ounces fresh baby spinach, chopped
- 3 cups vegetable broth
- 1/2 cup canned coconut milk
- Salt and pepper

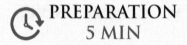 **PREPARATION**
5 MIN

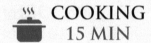 **COOKING**
15 MIN

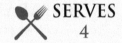 **SERVES**
4

DIRECTIONS

1. Heat the oil in a saucepan over medium-high heat – add the onion and garlic.
2. Sauté for 4 to 5 minutes until browned, then stir in the cauliflower.
3. Cook for 5 minutes until browned, and then stir in the spinach.
4. Let it cook for 2 minutes until wilted, then stir in the broth and bring to boil.
5. Remove from heat and puree the soup with an immersion blender.
6. Stir in the coconut milk and season with salt and pepper to taste. Serve hot.

Nutritions:

Calories: 165 kcal
Fat: 12 g
Protein: 7 g

Carbs: 9 g
Fiber: 2.5 g

76. EASY CHOPPED SALAD

INGREDIENTS

- 4 cups fresh chopped lettuce
- 1 small avocado, pitted and chopped
- 1/2 cup cherry tomatoes, halved
- 1/4 cup diced cucumber
- 2 hardboiled eggs, peeled and sliced
- 1 cup diced ham
- 1/2 cup shredded cheddar cheese

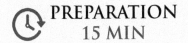 **PREPARATION** 15 MIN   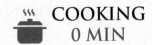 **COOKING** 0 MIN   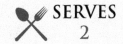 **SERVES** 2

DIRECTIONS

1. Divide the lettuce between two salad plates or bowls.
2. Top the salads with diced avocado, tomato, and celery.
3. Add the sliced egg, diced ham, and shredded cheese.
4. Serve the salads with your favorite keto-friendly dressing.

Nutritions:

Calories: 520 kcal
Fat: 39.5 g
Protein: 27 g

Carbs: 17.5 g
Fiber: 9 g

77. THREE MEAT AND CHEESE SANDWICH

INGREDIENTS

- 1 large egg, separated
- Pinch cream of tartar
- Pinch salt
- 1 ounce cream cheese, softened
- 1 ounce sliced ham
- 1 ounce sliced hard salami
- 1 ounce sliced turkey
- 2 slices cheddar cheese

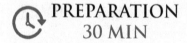 **PREPARATION** 30 MIN

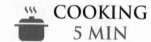 **COOKING** 5 MIN

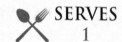 **SERVES** 1

DIRECTIONS

1. For the bread, preheat the oven to 305°f and line a baking sheet with parchment.
2. Beat the egg whites with the cream of tartar and salt until soft peaks form.
3. Whisk the cream cheese and egg yolk until smooth and pale yellow.
4. Fold in the egg whites a little at a time until it is smooth and well combined.
5. Spoon the batter onto the baking sheet into two even circles.
6. Bake for 25 minutes until firm and lightly browned.
7. To complete the sandwich, layer the sliced meats and cheeses between the two bread circles.
8. Grease a skillet with cooking spray and heat over medium heat.
9. Add the sandwich and cook until browned underneath then flips and cook until the cheese is melted.

Nutritions:

Calories: 610 kcal
Fat: 48 g
Protein: 40 g

Carbs: 3 g
Fiber: 0.5 g

78. BEEF AND PEPPER KEBABS

INGREDIENTS

- 2 tablespoons olive oil
- 1 1/2 tablespoon balsamic vinegar
- 2 teaspoons dijon mustard
- Salt and pepper
- 8 ounces beef sirloin, cut into 2-inch pieces
- 1 small red pepper, cut into chunks
- 1 small green pepper, cut into chunks

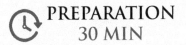 **PREPARATION**
30 MIN

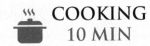 **COOKING**
10 MIN

 **SERVES**
2

DIRECTIONS

1. Whisk together the olive oil, balsamic vinegar, and mustard in a shallow dish.
2. Season the steak with salt and pepper, then toss in the marinade.
3. Let marinate for 30 minutes, and then slide onto skewers with the peppers.
4. Preheat a grill pan to high heat and grease with cooking spray.
5. Cook the kebabs for 2 to 3 minutes on each side until the beef is done.

Nutritions:

Calories: 365 kcal
Fat: 21.5 g
Protein: 35.5 g

Carbs: 6.5 g
Fiber: 1.5 g

79. CHICKEN FAJITA SOUP

INGREDIENTS

- 12 ounces chicken thighs
- 1 cup diced tomatoes
- 2 cups chicken stock
- 1/2 cup enchilada sauce
- 2 ounces chopped green chiles
- 1 tablespoon minced garlic
- 1 medium yellow onion, chopped
- 1 small red pepper, chopped
- 1 jalapeno, seeded and minced
- 2 teaspoons chili powder
- ¾ teaspoon paprika
- 1/2 teaspoon ground cumin

- Salt and pepper
- 1 small avocado, sliced thinly
- 1/4 cup chopped cilantro
- 1 lime, cut into wedges

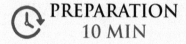 **PREPARATION**
10 MIN

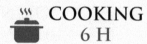 **COOKING**
6 H

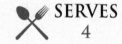 **SERVES**
4

DIRECTIONS

1. Combine the chicken, tomatoes, chicken stock, enchilada sauce, chiles, and garlic in the slow cooker and stir well.
2. Add the onion, bell peppers, and jalapeno.
3. Stir in the seasonings, then cover and cook on low for 5 to 6 hours.
4. Remove the chicken and chop or shred then stir it back into the soup.
5. Spoon into bowls and serve with sliced avocado, cilantro, and lime wedges.

Nutritions:

Calories: 325 kcal
Fat: 17 g
Protein: 28 g

Carbs: 17 g
Fiber: 7 g

80. AVOCADO EGG SALAD ON LETTUCE

INGREDIENTS

- 4 large hardboiled eggs, cooled and peeled
- 1 small avocado, pitted and chopped
- 1 medium stalk celery, diced
- 1/4 cup diced red onion
- 2 tablespoons fresh lemon juice
- Salt and pepper
- 4 cups chopped romaine lettuce

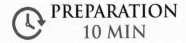 **PREPARATION**
10 MIN

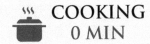 **COOKING**
0 MIN

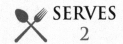 **SERVES**
2

DIRECTIONS

1. Coarsely chop the eggs into a bowl.
2. Toss in the avocado, celery, red onion, and lemon juice.
3. Season with salt and pepper then serve over chopped lettuce.

Nutritions:

Calories: 375 kcal
Fat: 30 g
Protein: 15.5 g

Carbs: 15 g
Fiber: 8 g

81. MEDITERRANEAN KETO DISH

INGREDIENTS

- 1 Roma tomato, halved
- 1/4 cup olive oil
- 2 ounces fresh mozzarella cheese, sliced
- 2 ounces tuna, packed in water
- 8 green olives

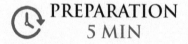 **PREPARATION**
5 MIN

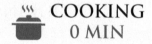 **COOKING**
0 MIN

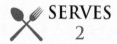 **SERVES**
2

DIRECTIONS

1. Take two serves plates and then distribute tomato, cheese, and tuna evenly between them.
2. Season with salt and black pepper and then serve with olive oil.

Nutritions:

Calories: 412 kcal
Fat: 35 g
Protein: 20 g

Carbs: 4 g
Fiber: 1.5 g

82. EASY ZUCCHINI NOODLES

INGREDIENTS

- 1 large zucchini, spiralized into noodles
- 2 tablespoons softened cream cheese
- 1 tablespoon grated parmesan cheese
- 1/8 teaspoon garlic powder

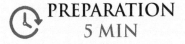 **PREPARATION**
5 MIN

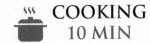 **COOKING**
10 MIN

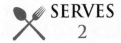 **SERVES**
2

DIRECTIONS

1. Prepare zucchini noodles, and for this, cut zucchini into noodles by using a spiralizer or a vegetable peeler.
2. Then bring out a skillet pan, place it over medium-high heat, add zucchini noodles and garlic, toss well until mixed, and cook for 4 minutes until slightly soft.
3. Push noodles to one side of the pan, add cream cheese into the other side of the pan, stir it until melts, then mix with noodles until coated and season with salt and black pepper.
4. Remove pan from heat, sprinkle zoodles with parmesan cheese and serve.

Nutritions:

Calories: 107 kcal
Fat: 9 g
Protein: 2 g

Carbs: 2 g
Fiber: 1 g

83. KETO CHEESE POTATO

INGREDIENTS

- 1 large turnip, peeled, diced
- 2 slices of bacon, chopped
- 1 tablespoon olive oil
- 1 tablespoon softened cream cheese
- 1/4 of spring onion, diced, and more for garnishing

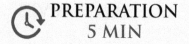 **PREPARATION** 5 MIN 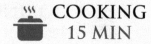 **COOKING** 15 MIN 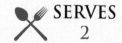 **SERVES** 2

DIRECTIONS

1. Bring out a skillet pan, place it over medium-high heat, add oil and when hot, add diced turnip, season with salt, black pepper, and paprika, sprinkle with garlic, stir well and cook for 5 minutes.
2. Then add onion, stir and continue cooking for 3 minutes until onions start to soften.
3. Add chopped bacon, continue cooking for 5 to 7 minutes or until bacon is crispy and remove the pan from heat.
4. Top with green onions and cream cheese and then serve.

Nutritions:

Calories: 88 kcal
Fat: 9 g
Protein: 3 g

Carbs: 3.5 g
Fiber: 1 g

84. CHICKEN PAN WITH VEGGIES AND PESTO

INGREDIENTS

- 2 Tbsp. olive oil
- 1 pound chicken thighs, boneless, skinless, sliced into strips
- ¾ cup oil-packed sun-dried tomatoes, chopped
- 1 pound asparagus ends
- 1/4 cup basil pesto
- 1 cup cherry tomatoes, red and yellow, halved
- Salt, to taste

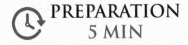 **PREPARATION** 5 MIN	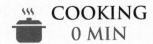 **COOKING** 0 MIN	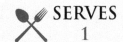 **SERVES** 1

DIRECTIONS

1. Heat olive oil in a frying pan over medium-high heat.
2. Put salt on the chicken slices and then put into a skillet, add the sun-dried tomatoes and fry for 5-10 minutes. Remove the chicken slices and season with salt. Add asparagus to the skillet. Cook for additional 5-10 minutes.
3. Place the chicken back in the skillet, pour in the pesto and whisk. Fry for 1-2 minutes. Remove from the heat. Add the halved cherry tomatoes and pesto. Stir well and serve.

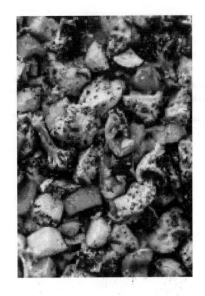

Nutritions:

Carbohydrates: 12 g
Fat: 32 g
Protein: 2 g

Calories: 423 kcal

85. CABBAGE SOUP WITH BEEF

INGREDIENTS

- 2 Tbsp. olive oil
- 1 medium onion, chopped
- 1 pound fillet steak, cut into pieces
- 1/2 stalk celery, chopped
- 1 carrot, peeled and diced
- 1/2 head small green cabbage, cut into pieces
- 2 cloves garlic, minced
- 4 cups beef broth
- 2 Tbsp. fresh parsley, chopped
- 1 tsp. dried thyme
- 1 tsp. dried rosemary
- 1 tsp. garlic powder
- Salt and black pepper, to taste

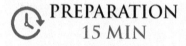 **PREPARATION** 15 MIN

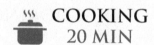 **COOKING** 20 MIN

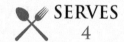 **SERVES** 4

DIRECTIONS

1. Heat oil in a pot (use medium heat). Add the beef and cook until it is browned. Put the onion into the pot and boil for 3-4 minutes.
2. Add the celery and carrot. Stir well and cook for about 3-4 minutes. Add the cabbage and boil until it starts softening. Add garlic and simmer for about 1 minute.
3. Pour the broth into the pot. Add the parsley and garlic powder. Mix thoroughly and reduce heat to medium-low.
4. Cook for 10-15 minutes.

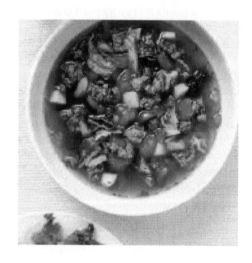

Nutritions:

Carbohydrates: 4 g
Fat: 11 g
Protein: 12 g

Calories: 177 kcal

86. CAULIFLOWER RICE SOUP WITH CHICKEN

INGREDIENTS

- 21/2 pounds chicken breasts, boneless and skinless
- 8 Tbsp. butter
- 1/4 cup celery, chopped
- 1/2 cup onion, chopped
- 4 cloves garlic, minced
- 2 12-ounce packages steamed cauliflower rice
- 1 Tbsp. parsley, chopped
- 2 tsp. poultry seasoning
- 1/2 cup carrot, grated
- ¾ tsp. rosemary

- 1 tsp. salt
- ¾ tsp. pepper
- 4 ounces cream cheese
- 4¾ cup chicken broth

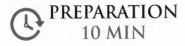 **PREPARATION**
10 MIN

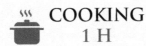 **COOKING**
1 H

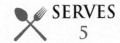 **SERVES**
5

DIRECTIONS

1. Put shredded chicken breasts into a saucepan and pour in the chicken broth. Add salt and pepper. Cook for 1 hour.
2. In another pot, melt the butter. Add the onion, garlic, and celery. Sauté until the mix is translucent. Add the riced cauliflower, rosemary, and carrot. Mix and cook for 7 minutes.
3. Add the chicken breasts and broth to the cauliflower mix. Put the lid on and simmer for 15 minutes.

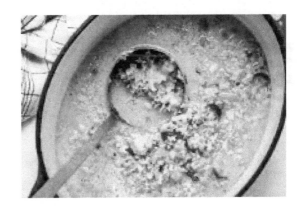

Nutritions:

Carbohydrates: 6 g
Fat: 30 g
Protein: 27 g

Calories: 415 kcal

87. QUICK PUMPKIN SOUP

INGREDIENTS

- 1 cup coconut milk
- 2 cups chicken broth
- 6 cups baked pumpkin
- 1 tsp. garlic powder
- 1 tsp. ground cinnamon
- 1 tsp. dried ginger
- 1 tsp. nutmeg
- 1 tsp. paprika
- Salt and pepper, to taste
- Sour cream or coconut yogurt, for topping
- Pumpkin seeds, toasted, for topping

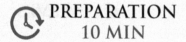 **PREPARATION** 10 MIN   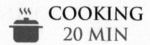 **COOKING** 20 MIN    **SERVES** 4-6

DIRECTIONS

1. Combine the coconut milk, broth, baked pumpkin, and spices in a soup pan (use medium heat). Stir occasionally and simmer for 15 minutes.
2. With an immersion blender, blend the soup mix for 1 minute.
3. Top with sour cream or coconut yogurt and pumpkin seeds.

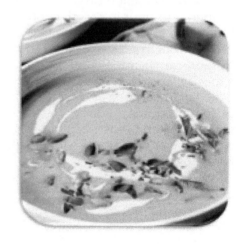

Nutritions:

Carbohydrates: 8.1 g   Calories: 123 kcal
Fat: 9.8 g
Protein: 3.1 g

88. FRESH AVOCADO SOUP

INGREDIENTS

- 1 ripe avocado
- 2 romaine lettuce leaves, washed and chopped
- 1 cup coconut milk, chilled
- 1 Tbsp. lime juice
- 20 fresh mint leaves
- Salt, to taste

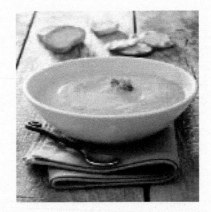

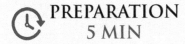 **PREPARATION** 5 MIN   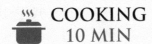 **COOKING** 10 MIN   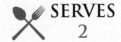 **SERVES** 2

DIRECTIONS

1. Mix all your ingredients thoroughly in a blender.
2. Chill in the fridge for 5-10 minutes.

Nutritions:

Carbohydrates: 12 g
Fat: 26 g
Protein: 4 g

Calories: 280 kcal

89. CREAMY GARLIC CHICKEN

INGREDIENTS

- 4 chicken breasts, finely sliced
- 1 tsp. garlic powder
- 1 tsp. paprika
- 2 Tbsp. butter
- 1 tsp. salt
- 1 cup heavy cream
- 1/2 cup sun-dried tomatoes
- 2 cloves garlic, minced
- 1 cup spinach, chopped

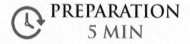 **PREPARATION**
5 MIN

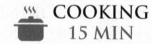 **COOKING**
15 MIN

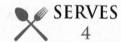 **SERVES**
4

DIRECTIONS

1. Blend the paprika, garlic powder, and salt and sprinkle over both sides of the chicken.
2. Melt the butter in a frying pan (choose medium heat). Add the chicken breast and fry for 5 minutes each side. Set aside.
3. Add the heavy cream, sun-dried tomatoes, and garlic to the pan and whisk well to combine. Cook for 2 minutes. Add spinach and sauté for an additional 3 minutes. Return the chicken to the pan and cover with the sauce.

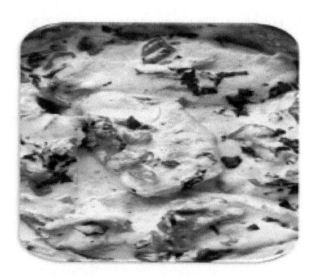

Nutritions:

Carbohydrates: 12 g
Fat: 26 g
Protein: 4 g

Calories: 280 kcal

90. CAULIFLOWER CHEESECAKE

INGREDIENTS

- 1 head cauliflower, cut into florets
- 1/3 cup sour cream
- 4 oz. cream cheese, softened
- 11/2 cup cheddar cheese, shredded
- 6 pieces bacon, cooked and chopped
- 1 tsp. salt
- 1/2 tsp. black pepper
- 1/4 cup green onion, chopped
- 1/4 tsp. garlic powder

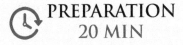 **PREPARATION** 20 MIN 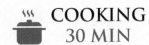 **COOKING** 30 MIN 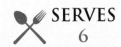 **SERVES** 6

DIRECTIONS

1. Preheat the oven to 350°F.
2. Boil the cauliflower florets for 5 minutes.
3. In a separate bowl combine the cream cheese and sour cream. Mix well and add the cheddar cheese, bacon pieces, green onion, salt, pepper, and garlic powder. Put the cauliflower florets into the bowl and combine with the sauce.
4. Put the cauliflower mix on the baking tray and bake for 15-20 minutes.

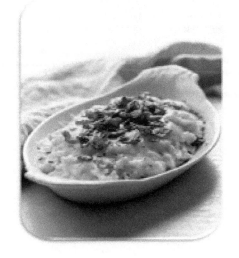

Nutritions:

Carbohydrates: 8 g
Fat: 26 g
Protein: 15 g

Calories: 320 kcal

91. CHINESE PORK BOWL

INGREDIENTS

- 1 1/4 pounds pork belly, cut into bite-size pieces
- 2 tbsp. tamari soy sauce
- 1 tbsp. rice vinegar
- 2 cloves garlic, smashed
- 3 oz. butter
- 1 pound Brussels sprouts, rinsed, trimmed, halved or quartered
- 1/2 leek, chopped
- Salt and ground black pepper, to taste

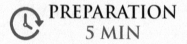 **PREPARATION** 5 MIN 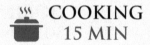 **COOKING** 15 MIN 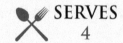 **SERVES** 4

DIRECTIONS

1. Fry the pork over medium-high heat until it is starting to turn golden brown.
2. Combine the garlic cloves, butter, and Brussels sprouts. Add to the pan, whisk well and cook until the sprouts turn golden brown.
3. Stir the soy sauce and rice vinegar together and pour the sauce into the pan.
4. Sprinkle with salt and pepper.
5. Top with chopped leek.

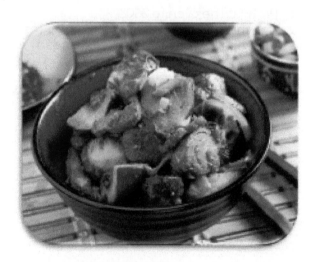

Nutritions:

Carbohydrates: 7 g
Fat: 97 g
Protein: 19 g

Calories: 993 kcal

92. TURKEY-PEPPER MIX

INGREDIENTS

- 1 pound turkey tenderloin, cut into thin steaks
- 1 tsp. salt, divided
- 2 tbsp. extra-virgin olive oil, divided
- 1/2 sweet onion, sliced
- 1 red bell pepper, cut into strips
- 1 yellow bell pepper, cut into strips
- 1/2 tsp. Italian seasoning
- 1/4 tsp. ground black pepper
- 2 tsp. red wine vinegar
- 1 14-ounces can crushed tomatoes, roasted
- Fresh parsley
- Basil

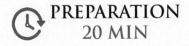 **PREPARATION** 20 MIN

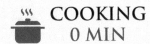 **COOKING** 0 MIN

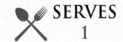 **SERVES** 1

DIRECTIONS

1. Sprinkle 1/2 tsp. salt on your turkey. Pour 1 Tbsp. oil into the pan and heat it. Add the turkey steaks and cook for 1-3 minutes per side. Set aside.
2. Put the onion, bell peppers, and the remaining salt to the pan and cook for 7 minutes, stirring all the time. Sprinkle with Italian seasoning and add black pepper. Cook for 30 seconds. Add the tomatoes and vinegar and fry the mix for about 20 seconds.
3. Return the turkey to the pan and pour the sauce over it. Simmer for 2-3 minutes.
4. Top with chopped parsley and basil.

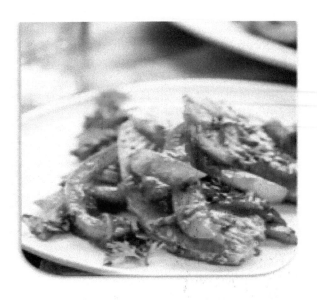

Nutritions:

Carbohydrates: 11 g
Fat: 8 g
Protein: 30 g

Calories: 230 kcal

93. SHRIMP SCAMPI WITH GARLIC

INGREDIENTS

- 1 pound shrimp
- 3 Tbsp. olive oil
- 1 bulb shallot, sliced
- 4 cloves garlic, minced
- 1/2 cup Pinot Grigio
- 4 Tbsp. salted butter
- 1 Tbsp. lemon juice
- 1/2 tsp. sea salt
- 1/4 tsp. black pepper
- 1/4 tsp. red pepper flakes
- 1/4 cup parsley, chopped

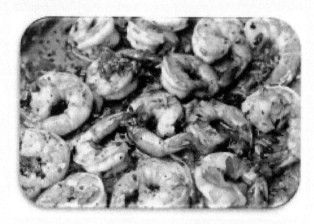

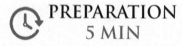 **PREPARATION** 5 MIN	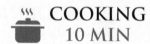 **COOKING** 10 MIN	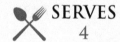 **SERVES** 4

DIRECTIONS

1. Pour the olive oil into the previously heated frying pan. Add the garlic and shallots and fry for about 2 minutes.
2. Combine the Pinot Grigio, salted butter, and lemon juice. Pour this mix into the pan and cook for 5 minutes.
3. Put the parsley, black pepper, red pepper flakes, and sea salt into the pan and whisk well.
4. Add the shrimp and fry until they are pink (about 3 minutes).

Nutritions:

Carbohydrates: 7 g
Fat: 7 g
Protein: 32 g

Calories: 344 kcal

94. CUCUMBER SALAD WITH TOMATOES AND FETA

INGREDIENTS

- 2 cucumbers, diced
- 6 tomatoes, diced
- ¾ cup feta cheese, crumbled
- 1/2 white onion, chopped
- 1 clove garlic, minced
- 2 Tbsp. lime juice
- 2 Tbsp. parsley, chopped
- 2 Tbsp. dill, chopped
- 3 Tbsp. olive oil
- 3 Tbsp. red wine vinegar
- Salt and black pepper, to taste

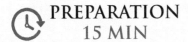 **PREPARATION** 15 MIN

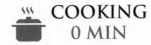 **COOKING** 0 MIN

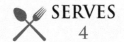 **SERVES** 4

DIRECTIONS

1. Combine all the ingredients in a bowl.
2. Stir thoroughly and serve.

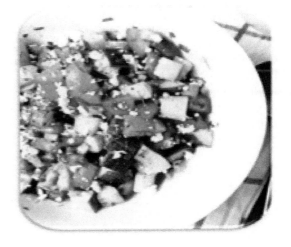

Nutritions:

Carbohydrates: 5 g
Fat: 10 g
Protein: 3 g

Calories: 125 kcal

95. CRAB CAKES WITH ALMOND FLOUR

INGREDIENTS

- 8 oz. fresh crab meat, shells removed
- 1 Tbsp. garlic, minced
- 1/4 cup parsley, chopped
- 1 egg, slightly beaten
- 1 Tbsp. avocado oil mayonnaise
- 1 Tbsp. mustard
- 1/2 tsp. kosher salt
- 1/2 tsp. dried thyme
- 1/8 tsp. cayenne pepper
- 1/2 cup almond flour
- 2 Tbsp. butter, for frying

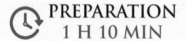 **PREPARATION** 1 H 10 MIN   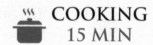 **COOKING** 15 MIN   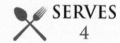 **SERVES** 4

DIRECTIONS

1. In a separate bowl, combine the crabmeat, garlic, parsley, egg, mayonnaise, mustard, kosher salt, thyme, cayenne pepper, and almond flour. Stir well. Form 4 cakes and place them into a fridge for 1 hour.
2. Melt the butter in the pan and put it in your crab cakes. Fry for about 5-7 minutes on each side.

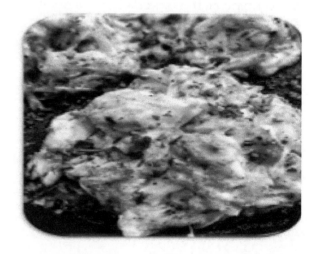

Nutritions:

Carbohydrates: 4 g   Calories: 219 kcal
Fat: 17 g
Protein: 13 g

96. STUFFED EGGS WITH BACON-AVOCADO FILLING

INGREDIENTS

- 2 eggs, boiled and halved
- 1 Tbsp. mayonnaise
- 1/4 tsp. mustard
- 1/8 lemon, squeezed
- 1/4 tsp. garlic powder
- 1/8 tsp. salt
- 1/8 tsp. smoked paprika
- 1/4 avocado
- 16 small pieces of bacon

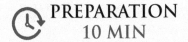 **PREPARATION**
10 MIN

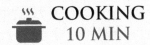 **COOKING**
10 MIN

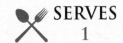 **SERVES**
1

DIRECTIONS

1. Fry the bacon for 3 minutes in a pan. Add the avocado and fry for an additional 3 minutes (lower heat).
2. Combine the mayonnaise, mustard, lemon, garlic powder, and salt in a separate bowl. Stir well.
3. Remove the yolk from the halved eggs and fill the egg halves with the mayonnaise mix. Top with the bacon-avocado filling.

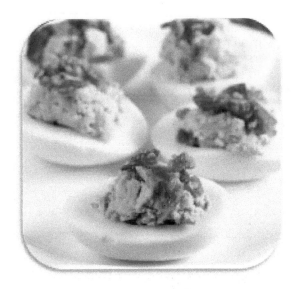

Nutritions:

Carbohydrates: 4 g
Fat: 30 g
Protein: 16 g

Calories: 342 kcal

97. SIMPLE TUNA SALAD

INGREDIENTS

- 10 oz. canned tuna, drained
- 1 avocado, chopped
- 1 rib celery, chopped
- 2 cloves fresh garlic, minced
- 3 Tbsp. mayonnaise
- 1 red onion, chopped
- Tbsp. lemon juice
- 8 sprigs parsley
- 1/4 cucumber, chopped
- Salt and pepper, to taste

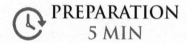 **PREPARATION** 5 MIN

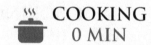 **COOKING** 0 MIN

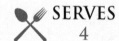 **SERVES** 4

DIRECTIONS

1. Divide the parsley into two halves.
2. Mix all the ingredients except half of the parsley in a separate bowl. Stir well.
3. Add salt and pepper to taste.
4. Top with the remaining parsley.

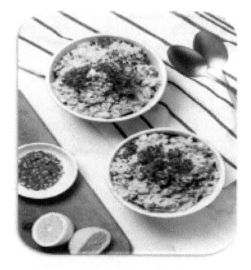

Nutritions:

Carbohydrates: 1.7 g   Calories: 225 kcal
Fat: 16.3 g
Protein: 13.9 g

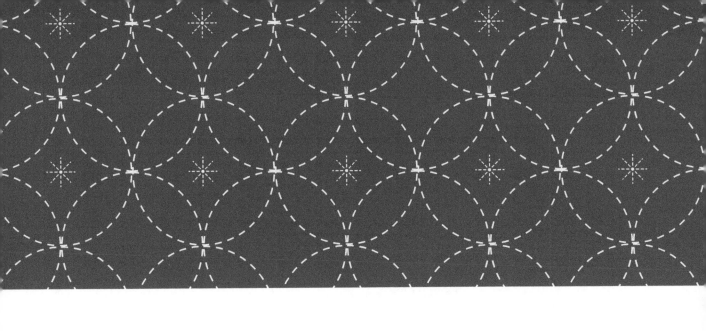

CHAPTER 8
APPETIZERS AND SNACKS

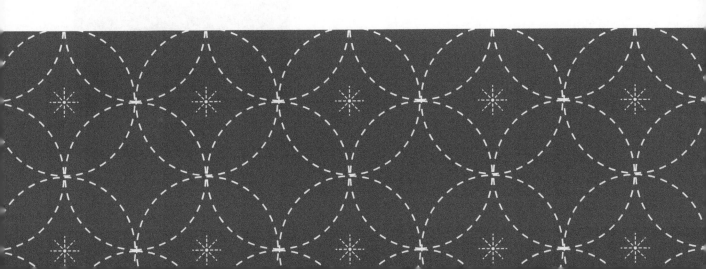

98. FRIED GREEN BEANS ROSEMARY

INGREDIENTS

- ¾ c. Green beans
- 3 tsp. Minced garlic
- 2 tbsps. Rosemary
- ½ tsp. Salt
- 1 tbsp. Butter

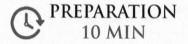 **PREPARATION** 10 MIN

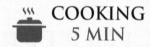 **COOKING** 5 MIN

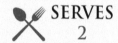 **SERVES** 2

DIRECTIONS

1. Warm-up an air fryer to 390°f.
2. Put the chopped green beans then brush with butter. Sprinkle salt, minced garlic, and rosemary over then cook within 5 minutes. Serve.

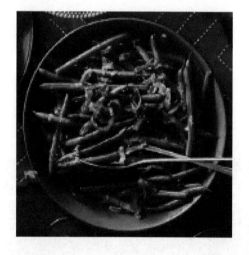

Nutritions:

Calories: 72 kcal
Fat: 6.3 g
Protein: 0.7 g

Carbs: 4.5 g

99. CRISPY BROCCOLI POP CORN

INGREDIENTS

- 2 c. Broccoli florets
- 2 c. Coconut flour
- 4 egg yolks
- ½ tsp. Salt
- ½ tsp. Pepper
- ¼ c. Butter

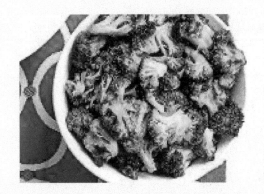

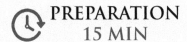 **PREPARATION**
15 MIN

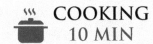 **COOKING**
10 MIN

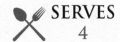 **SERVES**
4

DIRECTIONS

1. Dissolve butter, and then let it cool. Break the eggs in it.
2. Put coconut flour into the liquid, then put salt and pepper. Mix.
3. Warm-up an air fryer to 400°f.
4. Dip a broccoli floret in the coconut flour mixture, and then place it in the air fryer.
5. Cook the broccoli florets for 6 minutes. Serve.

Nutritions:

Calories: 202 kcal
Fat: 17.5 g
Protein: 5.1 g

Carbs: 7.8 g

100. CHEESY CAULIFLOWER CROQUETTES

INGREDIENTS

- 2 c. Cauliflower florets
- 2 tsp. Garlic
- ½ c. Onion
- ¾ tsp. Mustard
- ½ tsp. Salt
- ½ tsp. Pepper
- 2 tbsps. Butter
- ¾ c. Cheddar cheese

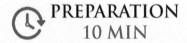 **PREPARATION** 10 MIN
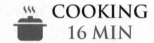 **COOKING** 16 MIN
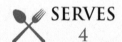 **SERVES** 4

DIRECTIONS

1. Microwave the butter. Let it cool.
2. Process the cauliflower florets using a processor. Transfer to a bowl then put chopped onion and cheese.
3. Put minced garlic, mustard, salt, and pepper, then pour melted butter over. Shape the cauliflower batter into medium balls.
4. Warm-up an air fryer to 400°f and cook within 14 minutes. Serve.

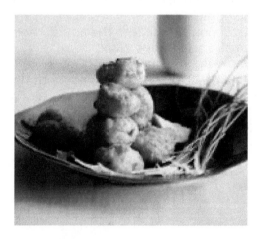

Nutritions:

Calories: 160 kcal
Fat: 13 g
Protein: 6.8 g

Carbs: 5.1 g

101. SPINACH IN CHEESE ENVELOPES

INGREDIENTS

- 3 c. Cream cheese
- 1½ c. Coconut flour
- 3 egg yolks
- 2 eggs
- ½ c. Cheddar cheese
- 2 c. Steamed spinach
- ¼ tsp. Salt
- ½ tsp. Pepper
- ¼ c. Onion

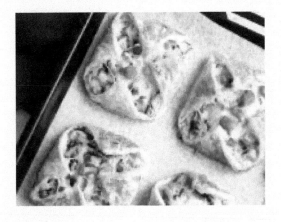

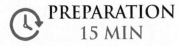 **PREPARATION**
15 MIN

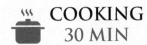 **COOKING**
30 MIN

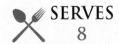 **SERVES**
8

DIRECTIONS

1. Whisk cream cheese put egg yolks. Stir in coconut flour until becoming soft dough.
2. Put the dough on a flat surface then roll until thin. Cut the thin dough into 8 squares.
3. Beat the eggs, and then place them in a bowl. Put salt, pepper, and grated cheese.
4. Put chopped spinach and onion into the egg batter.
5. Put spinach filling on a square dough then fold until becoming an envelope. Glue with water.
6. Warm-up an air fryer to 425°f (218°c). Cook within 12 minutes.
7. Remove and serve!

Nutritions:

Calories: 365 kcal   Carbs: 4.4 g
Fat: 34.6 g
Protein: 10.4 g

102. CHEESY MUSHROOM SLICES

INGREDIENTS

- 2 c. Mushrooms
- 2 eggs
- ¾ c. Almond flour
- ½ c. Cheddar cheese
- 2 tbsps. Butter
- ½ tsp. Pepper
- ¼ tsp. Salt

PREPARATION
8-10 MIN

COOKING
15 MIN

SERVES
8

DIRECTIONS

1. Processes chopped mushrooms in a food processor then add eggs, almond flour, and cheddar cheese.
2. Put salt and pepper then pour melted butter into the food processor. Transfer.
3. Warm-up an air fryer to 375°f (191°c).
4. Put the loaf pan on the air fryer's rack then cook within 15 minutes. Slice and serve.

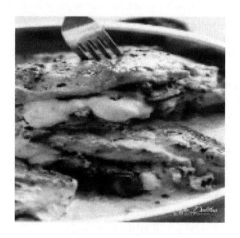

Nutritions:

Calories: 365 kcal   Carbs: 4.4 g
Fat: 34.6 g
Protein: 10.4 g

103. ASPARAGUS FRIES

INGREDIENTS

- Organic asparagus spears – 10
- Organic roasted red pepper– 1 tablespoon
- Almond flour – ¼ cup
- Garlic powder – ½ teaspoon
- Smoked paprika – ½ teaspoon
- Parsley – 2 tablespoons
- Parmesan cheese, and full-fat – ½ cup
- Organic eggs– 2
- Mayonnaise, full-fat – 3 tablespoons

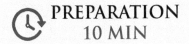 **PREPARATION** 10 MIN

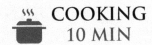 **COOKING** 10 MIN

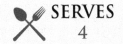 **SERVES** 4

DIRECTIONS

1. Warm-up oven to 425 degrees f.
2. Process cheese in a food processor, add garlic and parsley and pulse for 1 minute.
3. Add almond flour, pulse for 30 seconds, transfer and put paprika.
4. Whisk eggs into a shallow dish.
5. Dip asparagus spears into the egg batter, then coat with parmesan mixture and place it on a baking sheet. Bake in the oven within 10 minutes.
6. Put the mayonnaise in a bowl; add red pepper and whisk, and then chill. Serve with prepared dip.

Nutritions:

Calories: 453 kcal   Net Carbs: 5.5 g
Fat: 33.4 g
Protein: 19.1 g

104. KALE CHIPS

INGREDIENTS

- Organic kale – 1
- Seasoned salt – 1 tablespoon
- Olive oil – 2 tablespoons

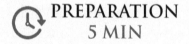 **PREPARATION** 5 MIN

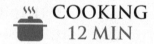 **COOKING** 12 MIN

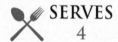 **SERVES** 4

DIRECTIONS

1. Warm-up oven to 350 degrees f.
2. Put kale leaves into a large plastic bag and add oil. Shake and then spread on a large baking sheet.
3. Bake within 12 minutes. Serve with salt.

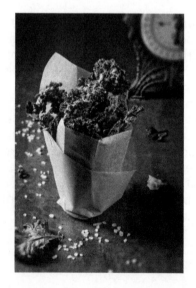

Nutritions:

Calories: 163 kcal
Fat: 10 g
Protein: 2 g

Net Carbs: 14 g

105. GUACAMOLE

INGREDIENTS

- Organic avocados pitted – 2
- Organic red onion – 1/3
- Organic jalapeño – 1
- Salt – ½ teaspoon
- Ground pepper – ½ teaspoon
- Tomato salsa – 2 tablespoons
- Lime juice – 1 tablespoon
- Organic cilantro – ½

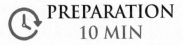 **PREPARATION**
10 MIN

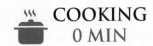 **COOKING**
0 MIN

 **SERVES**
4

DIRECTIONS

1. Slice the avocado flesh horizontally and vertically.
2. Mix in onion, jalapeno, and lime juice in a bowl.
3. Put salt and black pepper, add salsa and mix. Fold in cilantro and serve.

Nutritions:

Calories: 16.5 kcal
Fat: 1.4 g
Protein: 0.23 g

Net Carbs: 0.5 g

106. ZUCCHINI NOODLES

INGREDIENTS

- Zucchini, spiralized into noodles – 2
- Butter, unsalted – 2 tablespoons
- Garlic – 1 ½ tablespoon
- Parmesan cheese– 3/4 cup
- Sea salt – ½ teaspoon
- Ground black pepper – ¼ teaspoon
- Red chili flakes – ¼ teaspoon

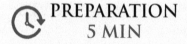 **PREPARATION**
5 MIN

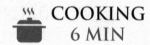 **COOKING**
6 MIN

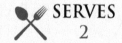 **SERVES**
2

DIRECTIONS

1. Sauté butter and garlic within 1 minute.
2. Put zucchini noodles, cook within 5 minutes, then put salt and black pepper.
3. Transfer then top with cheese and sprinkle with red chili flakes. Serve.

Nutritions:

Calories: 298 kcal
Fat: 26.1 g
Protein: 5 g

Net Carbs: 2.3 g
Fiber: 0.1 g

107. CAULIFLOWER SOUFFLÉ

INGREDIENTS

- Cauliflower, florets – 1
- Eggs – 2
- Heavy cream – 2 tablespoons
- Cream cheese – 2 ounces
- Sour cream – 1/2 cup
- Asiago cheese – 1/2 cup
- Cheddar cheese – 1 cup
- Chives – ¼ cup
- Butter, unsalted – 2 tablespoons
- Bacon, sugar-free – 6
- Water – 1 cup

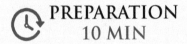 **PREPARATION** 10 MIN   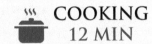 **COOKING** 12 MIN   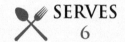 **SERVES** 6

DIRECTIONS

1. Pulse eggs, heavy cream, sour cream, cream cheese, and cheeses in a food processor.
2. Put cauliflower florets, pulse for 2 seconds, and then add butter and chives and pulse for another 2 seconds.
3. Put in water in a pot, and insert a trivet stand.
4. Put the cauliflower batter in a greased round casserole dish then put the dish on the trivet stand.
5. Cook within 12 minutes at high. Remove, top with bacon, and serve.

Nutritions:

Calories: 342 kcal   Net Carbs: 5 g
Fat: 28 g
Protein: 17 g

108. BANANA WAFFLES

INGREDIENTS

- 4 eggs
- 1 ripe banana
- ¾ cup coconut milk
- ¾ cup almond flour
- 1 pinch of salt
- 1 tbsp. of ground psyllium husk powder
- 1/2 tsp. vanilla extract
- 1 tsp. baking powder
- 1 tsp. of ground cinnamon
- Butter or coconut oil for frying

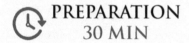 **PREPARATION**
30 MIN

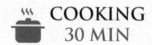 **COOKING**
30 MIN

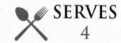 **SERVES**
4

DIRECTIONS

1. Mash the banana thoroughly until you get a mashed potato consistency.
2. Add all the other ingredients in and whisk thoroughly to evenly distribute the dry and wet ingredients. You should be able to get a pancake-like consistency
3. Fry the waffles in a pan or use a waffle maker.
4. You can serve it with hazelnut spread and fresh berries. Enjoy!

Nutritions:

Each Waffle Contains:

Carbohydrates: 4g

Fat: 13g

Protein: 5g

Calories: 155 kcal

109. KETO CINNAMON COFFEE

INGREDIENTS

- 2 tbsp. ground coffee
- 1/3 cup heavy whipping cream
- 1 tsp. ground cinnamon
- 2 cups water

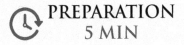 **PREPARATION**
5 MIN

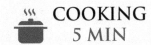 **COOKING**
5 MIN

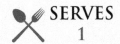 **SERVES**
1

DIRECTIONS

1. Start by mixing the cinnamon with the ground coffee.
2. Pour in hot water and do what you usually do when brewing.
3. Use a mixer or whisk to whip the cream 'til you get stiff peaks
4. Serve in a tall mug and put the whipped cream on the surface. Sprinkle with some cinnamon and enjoy.

Nutritions:

Net Carbs: 1 g
Fiber: 1 g
Fat: 14 g

Protein: 1 g
Calories: 136 kcal

110. KETO WAFFLES AND BLUEBERRIES

INGREDIENTS

- 8 eggs
- 5 oz. melted butter
- 1 tsp. vanilla extract
- 2 tsp. baking powder
- 1/3 cup coconut flour
- 3 oz. butter (topping)
- 1 oz. fresh blueberries (topping)

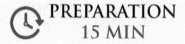 **PREPARATION**
15 MIN

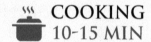 **COOKING**
10-15 MIN

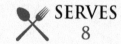 **SERVES**
8

DIRECTIONS

1. Start by mixing the butter and eggs first until you get a smooth batter. Put in the remaining ingredients except those that we'll be using as topping.
2. Heat your waffle iron to medium temperature and start pouring in the batter for cooking
3. In a separate bowl, mix the butter and blueberries using a hand mixer. Use this to top off your freshly cooked waffles.

Nutritions:

Net Carbs: 3 g
Fiber: 5 g
Fat: 56 g

Protein: 14 g
Calories: 575 kcal

111. MUSHROOM OMELET

INGREDIENTS

- 3 eggs, medium
- 1 oz. shredded cheese
- 1 oz. butter used for frying
- 1/4 yellow onion, chopped
- 4 large sliced mushrooms
- Your favorite vegetables, optional
- Salt and pepper to taste

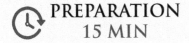 **PREPARATION**
15 MIN

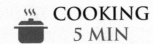 **COOKING**
5 MIN

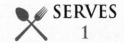 **SERVES**
1

DIRECTIONS

1. Crack and whisk the eggs in a bowl. Add some salt and pepper to taste.
2. Melt the butter in a pan using low heat. Put in the mushroom and onion, cooking the two until you get that amazing smell.
3. Pour the egg mix into the pan and allow it to cook on medium heat.
4. Allow the bottom part to cook before sprinkling the cheese on top of the still-raw portion of the egg.
5. Carefully pry the edges of the omelet and fold it in half. Allow it to cook for a few more seconds before removing the pan from the heat and sliding it directly onto your plate.

Nutritions:

Carbohydrates: 5 g
Fiber: 1 g
Fat: 44 g

Protein: 26 g
Calories: 520 kcal

112. CHOCOLATE SEA SALT SMOOTHIE

INGREDIENTS

- 1 avocado (frozen or not)
- 2 cups almond milk
- 1tbsp tahini
- 1/4 cup cocoa powder
- 1 scoop perfect Keto chocolate base

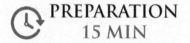 **PREPARATION** 15 MIN 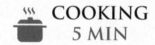 **COOKING** 5 MIN 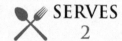 **SERVES** 2

DIRECTIONS

1. Combine all the ingredients in a high-speed blender and mix until you get a soft smoothie.
2. Add ice and enjoy!

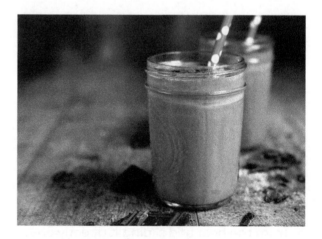

Nutritions:

Calories: 235 kcal
Fat: 20 g
Carbohydrates: 11.25 g

Fiber: 8 g
Protein: 5.5 g

113. ZUCCHINI LASAGNA

INGREDIENTS

- 3 cups raw macadamia nuts or soaked blanched almonds (for ricotta)
- 2 tbsp. Nutritional yeast (for ricotta)
- 2 tsp. dried oregano (for ricotta)
- 1 tsp. sea salt (for ricotta)
- 1/2 cup water or more as needed (for ricotta)
- 1/4 cup vegan parmesan cheese (for ricotta)
- 1/2 cup fresh basil, chopped (for ricotta)
- 1 medium lemon, juiced (for ricotta)
- Black pepper to taste (for ricotta)

- 1 28-oz jar favorite marinara sauce
- 3 medium zucchini squash thinly sliced with a mandolin

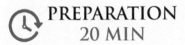 **PREPARATION** 20 MIN

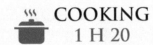 **COOKING** 1 H 20

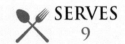 **SERVES** 9

DIRECTIONS

1. Preheat the oven to 375 degrees Fahrenheit
2. Put macadamia nuts into a food processor.
3. Add the remaining ingredients and continue to puree the mixture. You want to create a fine paste.
4. Taste and adjust the seasonings depending on your personal preferences.
5. Pour 1 cup of marinara sauce into a baking dish.
6. Start creating the lasagna layers using thinly sliced zucchini
7. Scoop small amounts of the ricotta mixture on the zucchini and spread it into a thin layer. Continue the layering until you've run out of zucchini or space for it.
8. Sprinkle parmesan cheese on the topmost layer.
9. Cover the pan with foil and bake for 45 minutes.
10. Remove the foil and bake for 15 minutes more.
11. Allow it to cool for 15 minutes before serving. Serve immediately.
12. The lasagna will keep for 3 days in the fridge.

Nutritions:

Calories: 338 kcal
Fat: 34 g
Carbohydrates: 10 g

Fiber: 5 g
Protein: 4.7 g

114. VEGAN KETO SCRAMBLE

INGREDIENTS

- 14 oz. firm tofu
- 3 tbsp. avocado oil
- 2 tbsp. yellow onion, diced
- 1.5 tbsp. Nutritional yeast
- 1/2 tsp. turmeric
- 1/2 tsp. garlic powder
- 1/2 tsp. salt
- 1 cup baby spinach
- 3 grape tomatoes
- 3 oz. vegan cheddar cheese

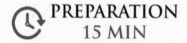 **PREPARATION** 15 MIN

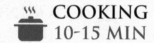 **COOKING** 10-15 MIN

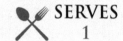 **SERVES** 1

DIRECTIONS

1. Start by squeezing the water out of the tofu block using a clean cloth or a paper towel.
2. Grab a skillet and put it on medium heat. Sauté the chopped onion in a small amount of avocado oil until it starts to caramelize
3. Using a potato masher, crumble the tofu on the skillet. Do this thoroughly until the tofu looks a lot like scrambled eggs.
4. Drizzle some more of the avocado oil onto the mix together with the dry seasonings. Stir thoroughly and evenly distribute the flavor.
5. Cook under medium heat, occasionally stirring to avoid burning of the tofu. You'd want most of the liquid to evaporate until you get a nice chunk of scrambled tofu.
6. Fold the baby spinach, cheese, and diced tomato. Cook for a few more minutes until the cheese melted. Serve and enjoy!

Nutritions:

Calories: 212 kcal
Fat: 17.5 g
Net Carbohydrates: 4.74 g

Protein: 10 g

115. PARMESAN CHEESE STRIPS

INGREDIENTS

- 1 cup shredded parmesan cheese
- 1 tsp. dried basil

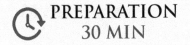 **PREPARATION**
30 MIN

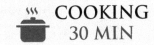 **COOKING**
30 MIN

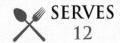 **SERVES**
12

DIRECTIONS

1. Preheat the oven to 350 degrees Fahrenheit. Prepare the baking sheet by lining it with parchment paper.
2. Form small piles of the parmesan cheese on the baking sheet. Flatten it out evenly and then sprinkle dried basil on top of the cheese.
3. Bake for 5 to 7 minutes or until you get a golden brown color with crispy edges. Take it out, serve, and enjoy!

Nutritions:

Calories: 31 kcal
Fat: 2 g
Protein: 2 g

116. PEANUT BUTTER POWER GRANOLA

INGREDIENTS

- 1 cup shredded coconut or almond flour
- 1 1/2 cups almonds
- 1 1/2 cups pecans
- 1/3 cup swerve sweetener
- 1/3 cup vanilla whey protein powder
- 1/3 cup peanut butter
- 1/4 cup sunflower seeds
- 1/4 cup butter
- 1/4 cup water

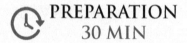 **PREPARATION** 30 MIN

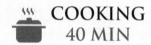 **COOKING** 40 MIN

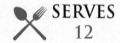 **SERVES** 12

DIRECTIONS

1. Preheat the oven to 300 degrees Fahrenheit and prepare a baking sheet with parchment paper
2. Place the almonds and pecans in a food processor. Put them all in a large bowl and add the sunflower seeds, shredded coconut, vanilla, sweetener, and protein powder.
3. Melt the peanut butter and butter together in the microwave.
4. Mix the melted butter in the nut mixture and stir it thoroughly until the nuts are well-distributed.
5. Put in the water to create a lumpy mixture.
6. Scoop out small amounts of the mixture and place it on the baking sheet.
7. Bake for 30 minutes. Enjoy!

Nutritions:

Calories: 338 kcal
Fat 30 g
Carbohydrates: 5 g

Protein: 9.6 g
Fiber: 5 g

117. HOMEMADE GRAHAM CRACKERS

INGREDIENTS

- 1 egg, large
- 2 cups almond flour
- 1/3 cup swerve brown
- 2 tsp. cinnamon
- 1 tsp. baking powder
- 2 tbsp. melted butter
- 1 tsp. vanilla extract
- Salt

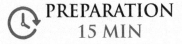 **PREPARATION**
15 MIN

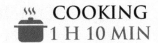 **COOKING**
1 H 10 MIN

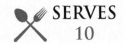 **SERVES**
10

DIRECTIONS

1. Preheat the oven to 300 degrees Fahrenheit
2. Grab a bowl and whisk the almond flour, cinnamon, sweetener, baking powder, and salt. Stir all the ingredients together.
3. Put in the egg, molasses, melted butter, and vanilla extract. Stir until you get a dough-like consistency.
4. Roll out the dough evenly, making sure that you don't go beyond 1/4 of an inch thick. Cut the dough into the shapes you want for cooking. Transfer it to the baking tray
5. Bake for 20 to 30 minutes until it firms up. Let it cool for 30 minutes outside of the oven and then put them back in for another 30 minutes. Make sure that for the second time putting the biscuit; the temperature is not higher than 200 degrees Fahrenheit. This last step will make the biscuit crispy.

Nutritions:

Calories: 156 kcal
Fat: 13.35 g
Carbohydrates: 6.21 g

Protein: 5.21 g
Fiber: 2.68 g

118. KETO NO-BAKE COOKIES

INGREDIENTS

- 2/3 cup all-natural peanut butter
- 1 cup all-natural shredded coconut, unsweetened
- 2 tbsp. real butter
- 4 drops of vanilla lakanto

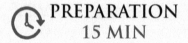 **PREPARATION** 15 MIN　　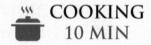 **COOKING** 10 MIN　　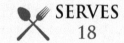 **SERVES** 18

DIRECTIONS

1. Melt the butter in the microwave.
2. Take it out and put in the peanut butter. Stir thoroughly.
3. Add the sweetener and coconut. Mix.
4. Spoon it onto a pan lined with parchment paper
5. Freeze for 10 minutes
6. Cut into preferred slices. Store in an airtight container in the fridge and enjoy whenever.

Nutritions:

Calories: 80 kcal

119. SWISS CHEESE CRUNCHY NACHOS

INGREDIENTS

- 1/2 cup shredded Swiss cheese
- 1/2 cup shredded cheddar cheese
- 1/8 cup cooked bacon pieces

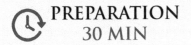
PREPARATION
30 MIN

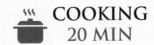
COOKING
20 MIN

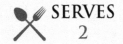
SERVES
2

DIRECTIONS

1. Preheat the oven to 300 degrees Fahrenheit and prepare the baking sheet by lining it with parchment paper.
2. Start by spreading the Swiss cheese on the parchment. Sprinkle it with bacon and then top it off again with the cheese.
3. Bake until the cheese has melted. This should take around 10 minutes or less.
4. Allow the cheese to cool before cutting them into triangle strips.
5. Grab another baking sheet and place the triangle cheese strips on top. Broil them for 2 to 3 minutes so they'll get chunky.

Nutritions:

Calories Per Serving: 280 kcal
Fat: 21.8 g

Protein: 18.6 g
Net Carbohydrates: 2.44 g

120. HEALTHY KETO GREEN SMOOTHIE

INGREDIENTS

- 1/2 cup coconut milk
- 1/2 cup chopped spinach
- 1/2 medium avocado, diced
- 1 tbsp. extra virgin coconut oil
- 1/2 tsp. vanilla powder
- 1/2 cup water
- A handful of ice cubes
- 1/4 cup chocolate whey protein
- 1 tsp. matcha powder
- 5 drops liquid stevia

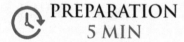 **PREPARATION** 5 MIN   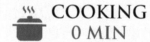 **COOKING** 0 MIN   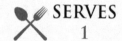 **SERVES** 1

DIRECTIONS

1. In a blender, combine all ingredients; blend until very smooth. Enjoy!

Nutritions:

Calories: 468 kcal
Total Fat: 48.3 g
Carbs: 6 g

Dietary Fiber: 4.5 g
Sugars: 1.2 g
Protein: 14.2 g

Cholesterol: 0 mg
Sodium: 109 mg

121. HEALTHY ZUCCHINI & BEEF FRITTATA

INGREDIENTS

- 1 tablespoon butter
- 1/2 red onion, minced
- 1 clove garlic, minced
- 8 ounces ground beef, crumbled
- 4 zucchinis, thinly sliced
- 6 free-range eggs
- Pinch of sea salt
- Pinch of pepper

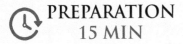 **PREPARATION** 15 MIN

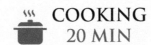 **COOKING** 20 MIN

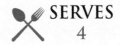 **SERVES** 4

DIRECTIONS

1. Preheat oven to 350°F.
2. Sauté red onion in an oven-safe skillet with butter for about 3 minutes or until tender;
3. Add garlic, beef, and zucchini and cook for about 7 minutes or until zucchini are tender and beef is cooked through.
4. Season with salt and pepper and remove from heat; cover the zucchini mixture with egg and bake for about 10 minutes or until the egg is set.
5. Serve warm.

Nutritions:

Calories: 263 kcal
Total Fat: 13.3 g
Carbs: 8.6 g

Dietary Fiber: 2.5 g
Sugars: 4.5 g
Protein: 28.1 g

Cholesterol: 304 mg;
Sodium: 229 mg

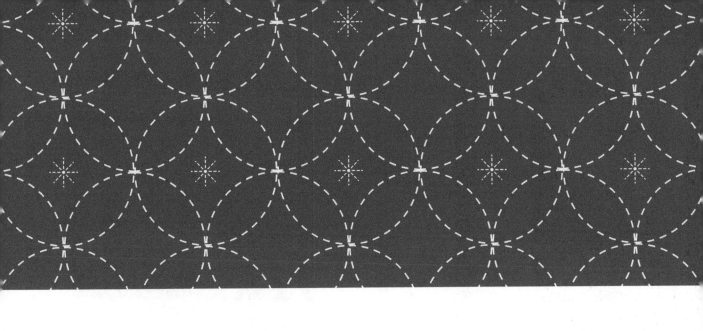

CHAPTER 9
FISH AND SEAFOOD

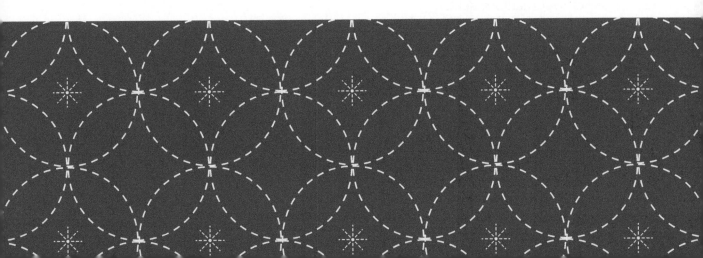

122. LEMONY SEA BASS FILLET

INGREDIENTS

- Fish:
- 4 sea bass fillets
- 2 tablespoons olive oil, divided
- A pinch of chili pepper
- Salt, to taste

Olive Sauce:
- 1 tablespoon green olives, pitted and sliced
- 1 lemon, juiced
- Salt, to taste

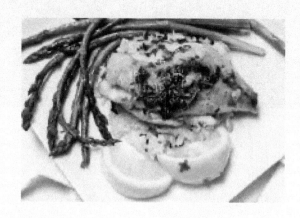

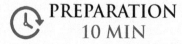 **PREPARATION** 10 MIN

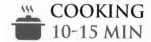 **COOKING** 10-15 MIN

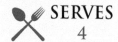 **SERVES** 4

DIRECTIONS

1. Preheat the grill to high heat.
2. Stir together one tablespoon olive oil, chili pepper, and salt in a bowl.
3. Brush both sides of each sea bass fillet generously with the mixture.
4. Grill the fillets on the preheated grill for about 5 to 6 minutes on each side until lightly browned.
5. Meanwhile, warm the left olive oil in a skillet over medium heat.
6. Add the green olives, lemon juice, and salt.
7. Cook until the sauce is heated through.
8. Transfer the fillets to four serving plates, then pour the sauce over them. Serve warm.

Nutritions:

Calories: 257 kcal
Fat: 12.4 g
Fiber: 56 g

Carbohydrates: 2 g
Protein: 12.7 g

123. CURRIED FISH WITH SUPER GREENS

INGREDIENTS

- 2 tablespoons coconut oil
- 2 teaspoons garlic, minced
- 1 1/2 tablespoons grated fresh ginger
- 1/2 teaspoon ground cumin
- 1 tablespoon curry powder
- 2 cups coconut milk
- ounces (454 g) firm white fish, cut into 1-inch chunks
- 1 cup kale, shredded
- 2 tablespoons cilantro, chopped

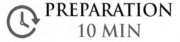 **PREPARATION** 10 MIN

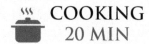 **COOKING** 20 MIN

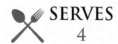 **SERVES** 4

DIRECTIONS

1. Melt the coconut oil in a heated pan
2. Add the garlic and ginger and sauté for about 2 minutes until tender.
3. Fold in the cumin and curry powder, then cook for 1 to 2 minutes until fragrant.
4. Put in the coconut milk and boil. Boil then simmer until the flavors mellow, about 5 minutes.
5. Add the fish chunks and simmer for 10 minutes until the fish flakes easily with a fork, stirring once.
6. Scatter the shredded kale and chopped cilantro over the fish, then cook for 2 minutes more until softened.

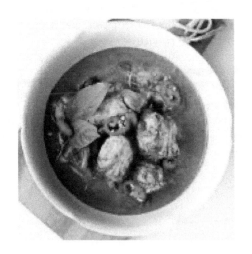

Nutritions:

Calories: 376 kcal
Fat: 19.9 g
Fiber: 15.8 g

Carbohydrates: 6.7 g
Protein: 14.8 g

124. SHRIMP ALFREDO

INGREDIENTS

- 1 pound of wild shrimp
- 3 tablespoons organic grass-fed whey
- 1 1/2 cups frozen asparagus
- 1 cup heavy cream
- 1/2 cup parmesan cheese
- Sea salt
- Black pepper
- 2 ground garlic cloves
- 1 small diced onion

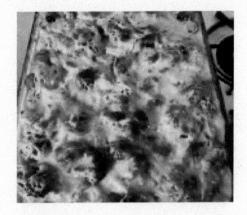

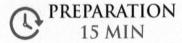 **PREPARATION**
15 MIN

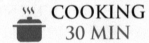 **COOKING**
30 MIN

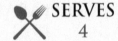 **SERVES**
4

DIRECTIONS

1. Peel and devein the shrimps, coat them well with salt and pepper. Let it cover in a bowl for 20 minutes.
2. Preheat a skillet. Put in butter, garlic, and onions.
3. When butter is melted, put in shrimp and stir fry till for 3 minutes.
4. Pour in heavy cream and stir well. Then, add ion cheese and stir till cheese melts.
5. Serve hot.

Nutritions:

Calories: 315 kcal
Fat: 11.9 g
Fiber: 8.5 g

Carbohydrates: 9.3 g
Protein: 11.1 g

125. GARLIC-LEMON MAHI MAHI

INGREDIENTS

- Tablespoons butter
- 5 tablespoons extra-virgin olive oil
- 4 ounces mahi-mahi fillets
- 3 minced cloves of garlic
- Kosher salt
- Black pepper
- 2 pounds of asparagus
- 2 sliced lemons
- Zest and juice of 2 lemons
- 1 teaspoon crushed red pepper flakes
- 1 tablespoon chopped parsley

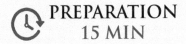 **PREPARATION** 15 MIN   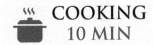 **COOKING** 10 MIN   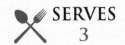 **SERVES** 3

DIRECTIONS

1. Melt three tablespoons of butter and olive oil in a microwave.
2. Heat a skillet and put in mahi-mahi, then sprinkle black pepper.
3. For around 5 minutes per side, cook it. When done, move to a plate.
4. In another skillet, add remaining oil and add in the asparagus, stir fry for 2-3 minutes. Take out on a plate.
5. In the same skillet, pour in the remaining butter, and add garlic, red pepper, lemon, zest, juice, and parsley.
6. Add in the mahi-mahi and asparagus and stir together. Serve hot.

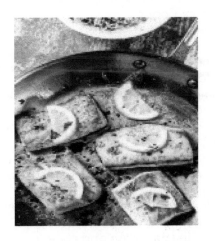

Nutritions:

Calories: 317 kcal
Fat: 8.5 g
Fiber: 6.9 g

Carbohydrates: 3.1 g
Protein: 16.1 g

126. SCALLOPS IN CREAMY GARLIC SAUCE

INGREDIENTS

- 11/4 pounds fresh sea scallops, side muscles removed
- Salt and ground black pepper, as required
- 4 tablespoons butter, divided
- garlic cloves, chopped
- 1/4 cup homemade chicken broth
- 1 cup heavy cream
- 1 tablespoon fresh lemon juice
- 2 tablespoons fresh parsley, chopped

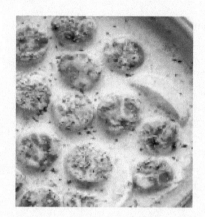

PREPARATION	COOKING	SERVES
15 MIN	15 MIN	4

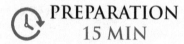 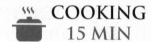 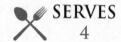

DIRECTIONS

1. Sprinkle the scallops evenly with salt and black pepper.
2. Melt two tablespoons of butter in a large pan over medium-high heat and cook the scallops for about 2–3 minutes per side.
3. Flip the scallops and cook for about two more minutes.
4. With a slotted spoon, transfer the scallops onto a plate.
5. Using the same pan, the butter must be melted and sauté the garlic for about 1 minute.
6. Pour the broth and bring to a gentle boil.
7. Cook for about 2 minutes.
8. Stir in the cream and cook for about 1–2 minutes or until slightly thickened.
9. Stir in the cooked scallops and lemon juice and remove from heat.
10. Garnish with fresh parsley and serve hot.

Nutritions:

Calories: 259 kcal
Fat: 8.5 g
Fiber: 7.4 g

Carbohydrates: 2.1 g
Protein: 12.2 g

127. SHRIMP CURRY

INGREDIENTS

- 2 tablespoons coconut oil
- 1/2 of yellow onion, minced
- 2 garlic cloves, minced
- 1 teaspoon ground turmeric
- 1 teaspoon ground cumin
- 1 teaspoon paprika
- 1 (14-ounce) can unsweetened coconut milk
- 1 large tomato, chopped finely
- Salt, as required
- 1-pound shrimp, peeled and deveined
- 2 tablespoons fresh cilantro, chopped

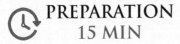 **PREPARATION** 15 MIN   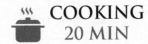 **COOKING** 20 MIN   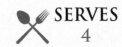 **SERVES** 4

DIRECTIONS

1. The coconut oil must be melted in a wok at medium heat and sauté the onion for about 5 minutes.
2. Add the garlic and spices, and sauté for about 1 minute.
3. Add the coconut milk, tomato, and salt, and bring to a gentle boil.
4. Let the curry simmer for about 10 minutes, stirring occasionally.
5. Stir in the shrimp and cilantro and simmer for about 4–5 minutes.

Nutritions:

Calories: 354 kcal
Fat: 12.5 g
Fiber: 7.5 g

Carbohydrates: 4.1 g
Protein: 14.1 g

128. ISRAELI SALMON SALAD

INGREDIENTS

- 1 cup flaked smoked salmon
- 1 tomato, chopped
- 1/2 small red onion, chopped
- 1 cucumber, chopped
- tbsp. pitted green olives
- 1 avocado, chopped
- 2 tbsp. avocado oil
- 2 tbsp. almond oil
- 1 tbsp. plain vinegar
- Salt and black pepper to taste
- 1 cup crumbled feta cheese
- 1 cup grated cheddar cheese

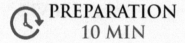 **PREPARATION** 10 MIN

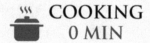 **COOKING** 0 MIN

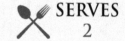 **SERVES** 2

DIRECTIONS

1. In a salad bowl, add the salmon, tomatoes, red onion, cucumber, green olives, and avocado. Mix well.
2. In a bowl, whisk the avocado oil, vinegar, salt, and black pepper.
3. Drizzle the dressing over the salad and toss well.
4. Sprinkle some feta cheese and serve the salad immediately.

Nutritions:

Calories: 415 kcal
Fat: 11.4 g
Fiber: 9.9 g

Carbohydrates: 3.8 g
Protein: 15.4 g

129. GREEK TUNA SALAD

INGREDIENTS

- 3 cans tuna
- 1/4 small red onion, finely chopped
- 1 celery stalks, finely chopped
- 1/2 avocado, chopped
- 1 tbsp. chopped fresh parsley
- 1 cup Greek yogurt
- 2 tbsp. butter
- 2 tsp. Dijon Mustard
- 1/2 tbsp. vinegar
- Salt and black pepper to taste

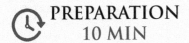 **PREPARATION**
10 MIN

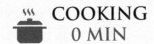 **COOKING**
0 MIN

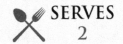 **SERVES**
2

DIRECTIONS

1. The ingredients listed must be added to a salad bowl and mix until well combined.
2. Serve afterward.

Nutritions:

Calories: 376 kcal
Fat: 10.4 g
Fiber: 11.9 g

Carbohydrates: 3.9 g
Protein: 18.4 g

130. BLACKENED SALMON WITH AVOCADO SALSA

INGREDIENTS

- 1 tbsp. extra virgin olive oil
- filets of salmon (about 6 oz. each)
- tsp. Cajun seasoning
- 2 med. avocados, diced
- 1 c. cucumber, diced
- 1/4 c. red onion, diced
- 1 tbsp. parsley, chopped
- 1 tbsp. lime juice
- Sea salt & pepper, to taste

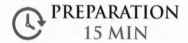 **PREPARATION**
15 MIN

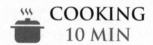 **COOKING**
10 MIN

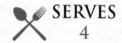 **SERVES**
4

DIRECTIONS

1. The oil must be heated in a skillet.
2. Rub the Cajun seasoning into the fillets, then lay them into the bottom of the skillet once it's hot enough.
3. Cook until a dark crust forms, then flip and repeat.
4. In a medium mixing bowl, combine all the ingredients for the salsa and set aside.
5. Plate the fillets and top with 1/4 of the salsa yielded.
6. Enjoy!

Nutritions:

Calories: 425 kcal
Fat: 15.8 g
Fiber: 19.2 g

Carbohydrates: 4.1 g
Protein: 11/8 g

131. TANGY COCONUT COD

INGREDIENTS

- 1/3 c. coconut flour
- 1/2 tsp. cayenne pepper
- 1 egg, beaten
- 1 lime
- 1 tsp. crushed red pepper flakes
- 1 tsp. garlic powder
- oz. cod fillets
- Sea salt & pepper, to taste

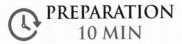 **PREPARATION**
10 MIN

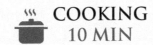 **COOKING**
10 MIN

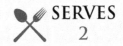 **SERVES**
2

DIRECTIONS

1. Let the oven preheat to 400°F/175°C. Then line a baking sheet with non-stick foil.
2. Place the flour in a shallow dish (a plate works fine) and drag the fillets of cod through the beaten egg. Dredge the cod in the coconut flour, then lay it on the baking sheet.
3. Sprinkle the fillet's top with the seasoning and lime juice.
4. Bake the cod for about 10 to 12 minutes until the fillets are flaky.
5. Serve immediately!

Nutritions:

Calories: 318 kcal
Fat: 12.1 g
Fiber: 15.1 g

Carbohydrates: 4.1 g
Protein: 19.5 g

132. FISH TACO BOWL

INGREDIENTS

- (5-ounce) tilapia fillets
- 1 tablespoon olive oil
- teaspoons Tajin seasoning salt, divided
- 2 cups pre-sliced coleslaw cabbage mix
- 1 tablespoon avocado mayo
- 1 tsp. hot sauce
- 1 avocado, mashed
- Pink Himalayan salt
- Freshly ground black pepper

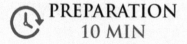 **PREPARATION** 10 MIN

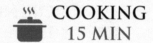 **COOKING** 15 MIN

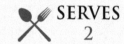 **SERVES** 2

DIRECTIONS

1. Preheat the oven to 425°F. The baking sheet must be lined with a baking mat.
2. Rub the tilapia with olive oil, and then coat it with two teaspoons of Tajín seasoning salt.
3. Place the fish in the prepared pan.
4. Let the tilapia bake for 15 minutes, or until the fish is opaque when you pierce it with a fork.
5. Meanwhile, in a medium bowl, gently mix to combine the coleslaw and the mayo sauce.
6. You don't want the cabbage super wet, just enough to dress it.
7. Add the mashed avocado and the remaining two teaspoons of Tajín seasoning salt to the coleslaw, and season with pink Himalayan salt and pepper.
8. Divide the salad between two bowls.
9. Shred fish into tiny pieces, and add them to the bowls.
10. Top the fish with a drizzle of mayo sauce and serve.

Nutritions:

Calories: 231 kcal
Fat: 12.1 g
Fiber: 10.3 g

Carbohydrates: 2.1 g
Protein: 17.3 g

133. SCALLOPS WITH CREAMY BACON SAUCE

INGREDIENTS

- Bacon slices
- 1 cup heavy (whipping) cream
- 1 tablespoon butter
- 1/4 cup grated Parmesan cheese
- Pink Himalayan salt
- Freshly ground black pepper
- 1 tablespoon ghee
- large sea scallops, rinsed and patted dry

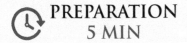 **PREPARATION** 5 MIN

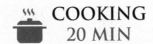 **COOKING** 20 MIN

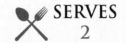 **SERVES** 2

DIRECTIONS

1. Cook the bacon.
2. Lower the heat to medium. Add the butter, cream, and Parmesan cheese to the bacon grease and season with a pinch of pink Himalayan salt and pepper.
3. Lower the heat down, then stir constantly until the sauce thickens and is reduced by 50 percent, about 10 minutes.
4. In another skillet, heat the ghee until sizzling.
5. Season the scallops with pink Himalayan salt and pepper, and add them to the skillet—Cook for just 1 minute per side.
6. Do not crowd the scallops; if your pan isn't large enough, cook them in two batches.
7. You want the scallops golden on each side.
8. Transfer the scallops to a paper towel-lined plate.
9. Divide the cream sauce between two plates, crumble the bacon on top of the cream sauce, and top with four scallops. Serve immediately.

Nutritions:

Calories: 311 kcal
Fat: 14.1 g
Fiber: 10.3 g

Carbohydrates: 1.2 g
Protein: 17.7 g

134. PARMESAN-GARLIC SALMON WITH ASPARAGUS

INGREDIENTS

- (6-ounce) salmon fillets, skin on
- Pink Himalayan salt
- Freshly ground black pepper
- 1-pound fresh asparagus ends snapped off
- tablespoons butter
- 2 garlic cloves, minced
- 1/4 cup grated Parmesan cheese

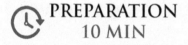 **PREPARATION**
10 MIN

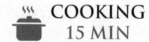 **COOKING**
15 MIN

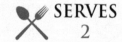 **SERVES**
2

DIRECTIONS

1. Oven: 400°F.
2. Pat the salmon dry and season both sides with pink Himalayan salt and pepper.
3. Put the salmon, and arrange the asparagus around the salmon.
4. Melt the butter. Add the minced garlic and stir until the garlic just begins to brown about 3 minutes.
5. Drizzle the garlic-butter sauce over the salmon and asparagus, and top both with the Parmesan cheese.
6. Bake until the salmon is cooked and the asparagus is crisp-tender, about 12 minutes. You can switch the oven to broil at the end of cooking time to char the asparagus.
7. Serve hot.

Nutritions:

Calories: 476 kcal
Fat: 14.1 g
Fiber: 10.5 g

Carbohydrates: 3.1 g
Protein: 19.9 g

135. SPICY SHRIMP SKEWERS

INGREDIENTS

- Tbsp. Paprika
- 1/2 tbsp. Onion powder
- 1/2 tbsp. dried thyme, crushed
- 1-pound shrimp, peeled and deveined
- 2 tbsp. Olive oil
- 1/2 tbsp. Red chili powder
- 1/2 tbsp. Garlic powder
- 1/2 tbsp. dried oregano, crushed
- 2 zucchinis, cut into 1/2-inch cubes

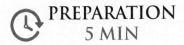 **PREPARATION** 5 MIN

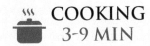 **COOKING** 3-9 MIN

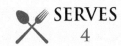 **SERVES** 4

DIRECTIONS

1. Preheat the grill to medium-high heat.
2. In a bowl, mix spices and dried herbs.
3. In a large bowl, add shrimp, zucchini, oil, and seasoning and toss to coat well.
4. Thread shrimp and zucchini onto pre-soaked skewers.
5. Grill the skewers for about 6-8 minutes, flipping occasionally. Serve hot.

Nutritions:

Calories: 261 kcal
Fat: 9.4 g
Fiber: 10.1 g

Carbohydrates: 3.2 g
Protein: 4.1 g

136. FRIED SHRIMP TAILS

INGREDIENTS

- 1-pound shrimp tails
- 1 tablespoon olive oil
- 1 teaspoon dried dill
- 1/2 teaspoon dried parsley
- 1 tablespoon coconut flour
- 1/2 cup heavy cream
- 1 teaspoon chili flakes

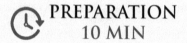 **PREPARATION** 10 MIN

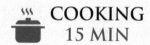 **COOKING** 15 MIN

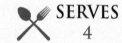 **SERVES** 4

DIRECTIONS

1. Peel the shrimp tails and sprinkle them with the dried dill and dried parsley.
2. Mix the shrimp tails carefully in the mixing bowl.
3. After this, combine the coconut flour, heavy cream, and chili flakes in a separate bowl and whisk it until you get the smooth batter.
4. Then preheat the air fryer to 330 F.
5. Transfer the shrimp tails in the heavy cream batter and stir the seafood carefully.
6. Then spray the air fryer rack and put the shrimp tails there.
7. Cook the shrimp tails for 7 minutes. After this, turn the shrimp tails into another side.
8. Cook the shrimp tails for 7 minutes more. When the seafood is cooked – chill it well. Enjoy!

Nutritions:

Calories: 212 kcal
Fat: 10.1 g
Fiber: 8.5 g

Carbohydrates: 2.6 g
Protein: 5.1 g

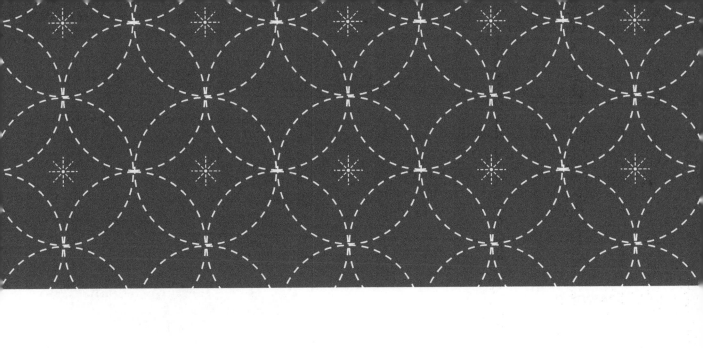

CHAPTER 10
MEAT

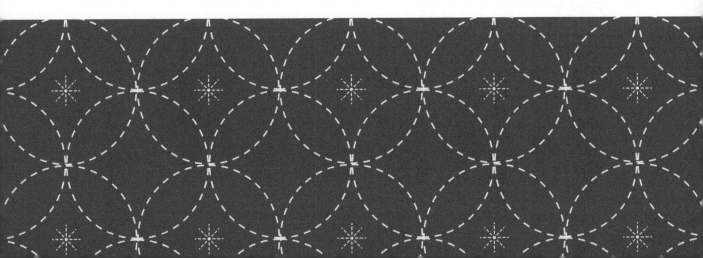

137. BEEF WITH CABBAGE NOODLES

INGREDIENTS

- 4 oz ground beef
- 1 cup chopped cabbage
- 4 oz tomato sauce
- ½ tsp minced garlic
- ½ cup water

Seasoning:
- ½ tbsp coconut oil
- ½ tsp salt
- ¼ tsp Italian seasoning
- 1/8 tsp dried basil

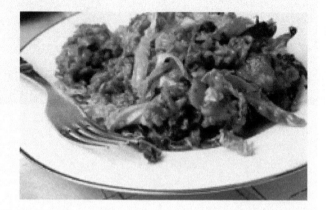

| 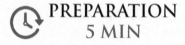 PREPARATION 5 MIN | 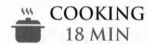 COOKING 18 MIN | 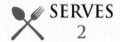 SERVES 2 |

DIRECTIONS

1. Take a skillet pan, place it over medium heat, add oil and when hot, add beef and cook for 5 minutes until nicely browned.
2. Meanwhile, prepare the cabbage and for it slice the cabbage into thin shred.
3. When the beef has cooked, add garlic, season with salt, basil, and Italian seasoning, stir well and continue cooking for 3 minutes until beef has thoroughly cooked.
4. Pour in tomato sauce and water, stir well and bring the mixture to boil.
5. Then reduce heat to medium-low level, add cabbage, stir well until well mixed and simmer for 3 to 5 minutes until cabbage is softened, covering the pan.
6. Uncover the pan and continue simmering the beef until most of the cooking liquid has evaporated.
7. Serve.

Nutritions:

Calories: 188.5 kcal
Fat: 12.5 g
Protein: 15.5 g

Net Carb: 2.5 g
Fiber: 1 g

138. ROAST BEEF AND MOZZARELLA PLATE

INGREDIENTS

- 4 slices of roast beef
- ½ ounce chopped lettuce
- 1 avocado, pitted
- 2 oz mozzarella cheese, cubed
- ½ cup mayonnaise

Seasoning:
- ¼ tsp salt
- 1/8 tsp ground black pepper
- 2 tbsp avocado oil

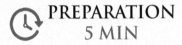 **PREPARATION** 5 MIN

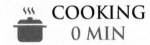 **COOKING** 0 MIN

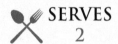 **SERVES** 2

DIRECTIONS

1. Scoop out flesh from the avocado and divide it evenly between two plates.
2. Add slices of roast beef, lettuce, and cheese and then sprinkle with salt and black pepper.
3. Serve with avocado oil and mayonnaise.

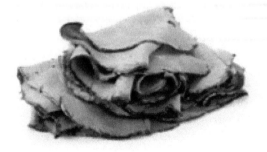

Nutritions:

Calories: 267.7 kcal
Fat: 24.5 g
Protein: 9.5 g

Net Carb: 1.5 g
Fiber: 2 g

139. BEEF AND BROCCOLI

INGREDIENTS

- 6 slices of beef roast, cut into strips
- 1 scallion, chopped
- 3 oz broccoli florets, chopped
- 1 tbsp avocado oil
- 1 tbsp butter, unsalted

Seasoning:
- ¼ tsp salt
- 1/8 tsp ground black pepper
- 1 ½ tbsp soy sauce
- 3 tbsp chicken broth

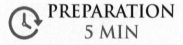 **PREPARATION 5 MIN**   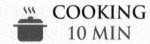 **COOKING 10 MIN**   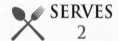 **SERVES 2**

DIRECTIONS

1. Take a medium skillet pan, place it over medium heat, add oil and when hot, add beef strips and cook for 2 minutes until hot.
2. Transfer beef to a plate, add scallion to the pan, then add butter and cook for 3 minutes until tender.
3. Add remaining ingredients, stir until mixed, switch heat to the low level, and simmer for 3 to 4 minutes until broccoli is tender.
4. Return beef to the pan, stir until well combined and cook for 1 minute.
5. Serve.

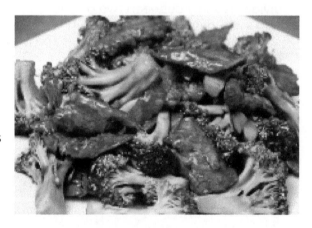

Nutritions:

Calories: 245 kcal
Fats: 15.7 g
Protein: 21.6 g

Net Carb: 1.7 g
Fiber: 1.3 g

140. GARLIC HERB BEEF ROAST

INGREDIENTS

- 6 slices of beef roast
- ½ tsp garlic powder
- 1/3 tsp dried thyme
- ¼ tsp dried rosemary
- 2 tbsp butter, unsalted

Seasoning:
- 1/3 tsp salt
- 1/4 tsp ground black pepper

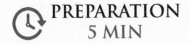 **PREPARATION**
5 MIN

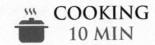 **COOKING**
10 MIN

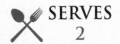 **SERVES**
2

DIRECTIONS

1. Prepare the spice mix and for this, take a small bowl, place garlic powder, thyme, rosemary, salt, and black pepper and then stir until mixed.
2. Sprinkle spice mix on the beef roast.
3. Take a medium skillet pan, place it over medium heat, add butter and when it melts, add beef roast and then cook for 5 to 8 minutes until golden brown and cooked.

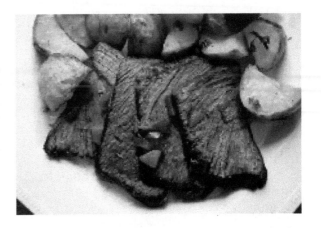

Nutritions:

Calories: 140 kcal
Fat: 12.7 g
Protein: 4.8 g

Net Carb: 1.7 g
Fiber: 2.6 g

141. SPROUTS STIR-FRY WITH KALE, BROCCOLI, AND BEEF

INGREDIENTS

- 3 slices of beef roast, chopped
- 2 oz Brussels sprouts, halved
- 4 oz broccoli florets
- 3 oz kale
- 1 ½ tbsp butter, unsalted
- 1/8 tsp red pepper flakes

Seasoning:
- ¼ tsp garlic powder
- ¼ tsp salt
- 1/8 tsp ground black pepper

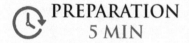 **PREPARATION** 5 MIN

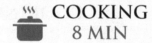 **COOKING** 8 MIN

 **SERVES** 2

DIRECTIONS

1. Take a medium skillet pan, place it over medium heat, add ¾ tbsp butter and when it melts, add broccoli florets and sprouts, sprinkle with garlic powder, and cook for 2 minutes.
2. Season vegetables with salt and red pepper flakes, add chopped beef, stir until mixed and continue cooking for 3 minutes until browned on one side.
3. Then add kale along with remaining butter, flip the vegetables and cook for 2 minutes until kale leaves wilts.
4. Serve.

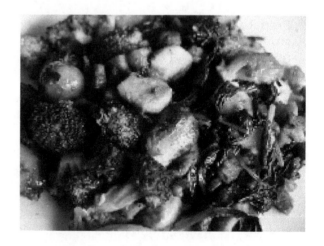

Nutritions:

Calories: 125 kcal
Fat: 9.4 g
Protein: 4.8 g

Net Carb: 1.7 g
Fiber: 2.6 g

142. BEEF AND VEGETABLE SKILLET

INGREDIENTS

- 3 oz spinach, chopped
- ½ pound ground beef
- 2 slices of bacon, diced
- 2 oz chopped asparagus

Seasoning:
- 3 tbsp coconut oil
- 2 tsp dried thyme
- 2/3 tsp salt
- ½ tsp ground black pepper

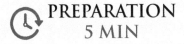 **PREPARATION**
5 MIN

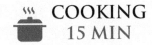 **COOKING**
15 MIN

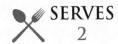 **SERVES**
2

DIRECTIONS

1. Take a skillet pan, place it over medium heat, add oil and when hot, add beef and bacon and cook for 5 to 7 minutes until slightly browned.
2. Then add asparagus and spinach, sprinkle with thyme, stir well and cook for 7 to 10 minutes until thoroughly cooked.
3. Season skillet with salt and black pepper and serve.

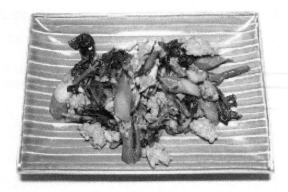

Nutritions:

Calories: 332.5 kcal
Fat: 26 g
Protein: 23.5 g

Net Carb: 1.5 g
Fiber: 1 g

143. BEEF, PEPPER AND GREEN BEANS STIR-FRY

INGREDIENTS

- 6 oz ground beef
- 2 oz chopped green bell pepper
- 4 oz green beans
- 3 tbsp grated cheddar cheese

Seasoning:
- ½ tsp salt
- ¼ tsp ground black pepper
- ¼ tsp paprika

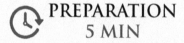 **PREPARATION** 5 MIN

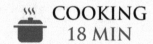 **COOKING** 18 MIN

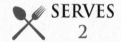 **SERVES** 2

DIRECTIONS

1. Take a skillet pan, place it over medium heat, add ground beef and cook for 4 minutes until slightly browned.
2. Then add bell pepper and green beans, season with salt, paprika, and black pepper, stir well and continue cooking for 7 to 10 minutes until beef and vegetables have cooked through.
3. Sprinkle cheddar cheese on top, then transfer pan under the broiler and cook for 2 minutes until cheese has melted and the top is golden brown.
4. Serve.

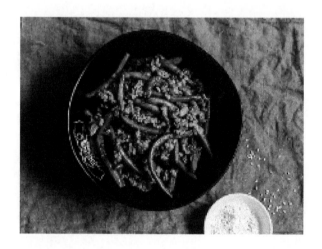

Nutritions:

Calories: 282.5 kcal
Fats: 17.6 g
Protein: 26.1 g

Net Carb: 2.9 g
Fiber: 1 g

144. CHEESY MEATLOAF

INGREDIENTS

- 4 oz ground turkey
- 1 egg
- 1 tbsp grated mozzarella cheese
- ¼ tsp Italian seasoning
- ½ tbsp soy sauce

Seasoning:
- ¼ tsp salt
- 1/8 tsp ground black pepper

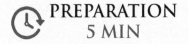 **PREPARATION** 5 MIN

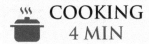 **COOKING** 4 MIN

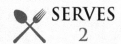 **SERVES** 2

DIRECTIONS

1. Take a bowl, place all the ingredients in it, and stir until mixed.
2. Take a heatproof mug, spoon in prepared mixture and microwave for 3 minutes at high heat setting until cooked.
3. When done, let meatloaf rest in the mug for 1 minute, then take it out, cut it into two slices and serve.

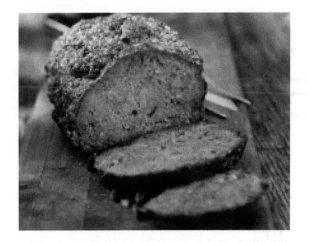

Nutritions:

Calories: 196.5 kcal
Fat: 13.5 g
Protein: 18.7 g

Net Carb: 18.7 g
Fiber: 0 g

145. ROAST BEEF AND VEGETABLE PLATE

INGREDIENTS

- 2 scallions, chopped into large pieces
- 1 ½ tbsp coconut oil
- 4 thin slices of roast beef
- 4 oz cauliflower and broccoli mix
- 1 tbsp butter, unsalted

Seasoning:
- 1/2 tsp salt
- 1/3 tsp ground black pepper
- 1 tsp dried parsley

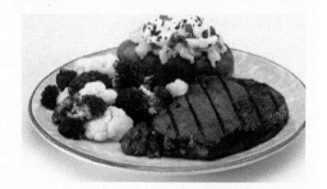

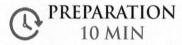 **PREPARATION** 10 MIN   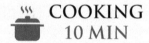 **COOKING** 10 MIN   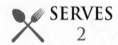 **SERVES** 2

DIRECTIONS

1. Turn on the oven, then set it to 400 degrees F, and let it preheat.
2. Take a baking sheet, grease it with oil, place slices of roast beef on one side, and top with butter.
3. Take a separate bowl, add cauliflower and broccoli mix, add scallions, drizzle with oil, season with remaining salt and black pepper, toss until coated and then spread vegetables on the empty side of the baking sheet.
4. Bake for 5 to 7 minutes until beef is nicely browned and vegetables are tender-crisp, tossing halfway.
5. Distribute beef and vegetables between two plates and then serve.

Nutritions:

Calories: 313 kcal
Fat: 26 g
Protein: 15.6 g

Net Carb: 2.8 g
Fiber: 1.9 g

146. STEAK AND CHEESE PLATE

INGREDIENTS

- 1 green onion, chopped
- 2 oz chopped lettuce
- 2 beef steaks
- 2 oz cheddar cheese, sliced
- ½ cup mayonnaise

Seasoning:
- ¼ tsp salt
- 1/8 tsp ground black pepper
- 3 tbsp avocado oil

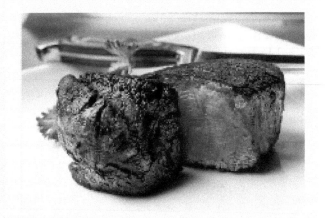

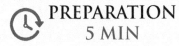 **PREPARATION**
5 MIN

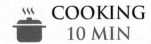 **COOKING**
10 MIN

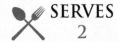 **SERVES**
2

DIRECTIONS

1. Prepare the steak, and for this, season it with salt and black pepper.
2. Take a medium skillet pan, place it over medium heat, add oil and when hot, add seasoned steaks and cook for 7 to 10 minutes until cooked to the desired level.
3. When done, distribute steaks between two plates, add scallion, lettuce, and cheese slices.
4. Drizzle with remaining oil and then serve with mayonnaise.

Nutritions:

Calories: 714 kcal   Net Carb: 4 g
Fat: 65.3 g   Fiber: 5.3 g
Protein: 25.3 g

147. GARLICKY STEAKS WITH ROSEMARY

INGREDIENTS

- 2 beef steaks
- 1/4 of a lime, juiced
- 1 ½ tsp garlic powder
- ¾ tsp dried rosemary
- 2 ½ tbsp avocado oil

Seasoning:
- ½ tsp salt
- ¼ tsp ground black pepper

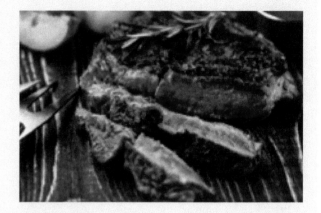

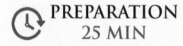 **PREPARATION**
25 MIN

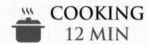 **COOKING**
12 MIN

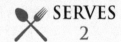 **SERVES**
2

DIRECTIONS

1. Prepare the steaks, and for this, sprinkle garlic powder on all sides of them.
2. Take a shallow dish, place 1 ½ tbsp oil and lime juice in it, whisk until combined, add steaks, turn to coat and let it marinate for 20 minutes at room temperature.
3. Then take a griddle pan, place it over medium-high heat and grease it with remaining oil.
4. Season marinated steaks with salt and black pepper, add to the griddle pan and cook for 7 to 12 minutes until cooked to the desired level.
5. When done, wrap steaks in foil for 5 minutes, then cut into slices across the grain.
6. Sprinkle rosemary over steaks slices and then serve.

Nutritions:

Calories: 213 kcal
Fat: 13 g
Protein: 22 g

Net Carb: 1 g
Fiber: 0 g

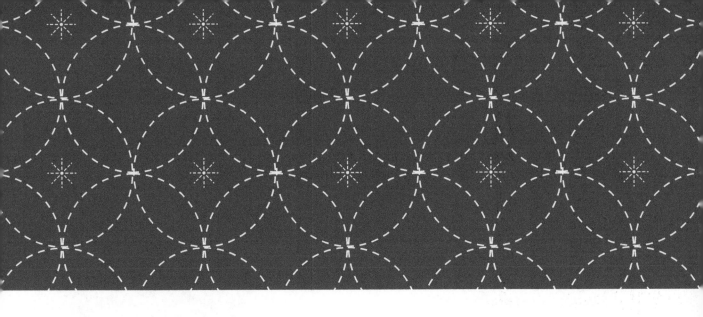

CHAPTER 11
SALADS AND VEGETABLES

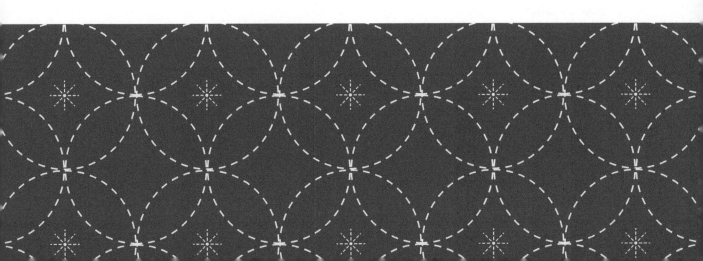

148. KETO COBB SALAD

INGREDIENTS

- 4 cherry tomatoes, diced
- 1 avocado, sliced
- 1 hardboiled egg, sliced
- 2 oz. chicken breast, shredded
- 1 oz. feta cheese, crumbled
- ¼ cup cooked bacon, crumbled
- 2 cups mixed green salad

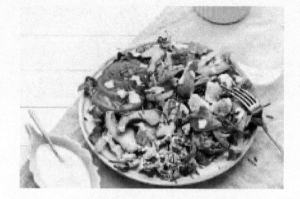

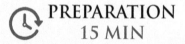 **PREPARATION**
15 MIN

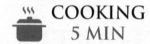 **COOKING**
5 MIN

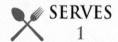 **SERVES**
1

DIRECTIONS

1. Mix the green salad in a large bowl. Add the chicken breast, feta cheese, and the crumbled bacon.
2. Put the tomatoes, avocado, egg, chicken, bacon, and feta cheese on top of the greens.
3. Enjoy! You can also try adding some ranch dressing but be aware that this adds to the total fat and calorie content of your salad.

Nutritions:

Calories: 412 kcal
Fat: 23.6 g
Cholesterol: 264.3 mg

Fiber: 6 g
Protein: 38.4 g

149. INGREDIENT KETO SALAD

INGREDIENTS

- 2 boneless chicken breasts with skin - 1 large avocado, sliced - 3 slices of bacon
- 4 cups mixed leafy greens of choice - 2 tbsp. dairy-free ranch dressing
- Salt and pepper to taste
- Duck fat for greasing

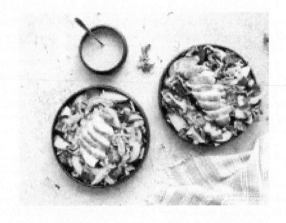

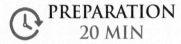 **PREPARATION**
20 MIN

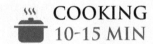 **COOKING**
10-15 MIN

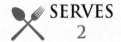 **SERVES**
2

DIRECTIONS

1. Start by preheating the oven to 200 degrees Celsius or 400 degrees Fahrenheit.
2. Season the chicken with salt and pepper. Grab a skillet and grease it with duck fat before cooking the chicken on the hot pan.
3. Keep the heat on high until you get a golden-brown skin surface. This should take around 5 minutes per side.
4. Once done, you can cook the chicken in the oven for 10 to 15 minutes. You can also put the bacon in with the chicken to save on the cooking time. You can also fry it in a pan, depending on your personal preferences.
5. After cooking, let the chicken rest for a few minutes.
6. Slice the avocado and the cooked chicken. Start assembling your salad, adding together the leafy greens, crispy bacon, sliced chicken, and avocado. Use 2 tablespoons of ranch dressing. Mix together until all ingredients are thoroughly coated. Enjoy!

Nutritions:

Carbs: 3.1 g
Protein: 38.7 g
Fat: 43.8 g

Calories: 581kcal

150. VEGETARIAN KETO COBB

INGREDIENTS

- 3 large hard-boiled eggs, sliced - 4 ounces cheddar cheese, cubed - 2 tbsp. sour cream
- 2 tbsp. mayonnaise - ½ tsp. garlic powder - ½ tsp. onion powder
- 1 tsp. dried parsley - 1 tbsp. milk - 1 tbsp. Dijon mustard
- 3 cups romaine lettuce, torn - 1 cup cucumber, diced
- ½ cup cherry tomatoes, halved

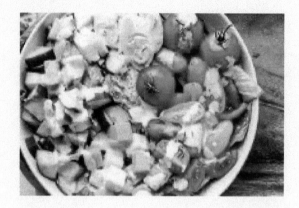

PREPARATION	COOKING	SERVES
10 MIN	0 MIN	3

DIRECTIONS

1. The dressing is a combination of the source cream, mayonnaise, and dried herbs. Mix them well together until fully combined.
2. Add one tablespoon of milk into the mix until you get the thickness you want.
3. Layer in the salad, adding all the ingredients that are not part of the dressing recipe. Put the mustard in the center of the salad.
4. Drizzle with your dressing and enjoy! Each serving should have just 2 tablespoons of dressing to meet the nutrition information given below.

Nutritions:

Calories: 330 kcal
Fat: 26.32 g
Protein: 16.82 g

Net carbohydrates: 4.83 g

151. KETO CHICKEN SALAD W/ AVOCADO

INGREDIENTS

- 2 pcs. of boneless chicken thigh fillets - 2 tbsp. olive oil - ¼ cup water
- 1 tsp. salt - 1 tsp. sweet chili powder - 1 tsp. dried thyme - ½ tsp. ground black pepper
- 4 cloves garlic - Handful of cherry tomatoes (salad) - 2 cups arugula (salad)
- 1 cup purslane leaves (salad) - ½ cup fresh dill (salad)
- 1 tbsp. olives (salad) - 1 tsp. sesame seeds (salad) - 1 tsp. nigella seeds (salad)
- ½ tbsp. olive oil (salad)

- 2 tbsp. avocado dressing (salad)
- 1 avocado, sliced (salad)
- Basil leaves (salad)

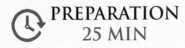 **PREPARATION** 25 MIN 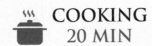 **COOKING** 20 MIN 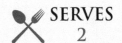 **SERVES** 2

DIRECTIONS

1. Pour ¼ cup of water on a skillet and cook the chicken fillets over medium heat, keeping the lid covered until the water drains completely.
2. Drizzle 2 tbsp. of olive oil on the chicken. Add some garlic cloves and then season it with salt and pepper. Add some thyme and sweet chili powder. Cook them again until golden, making sure you flip the chicken every now and again to even out the sides.
3. Put all ingredients in a bowl. Put in some nigella seeds and sesame seeds with some olive oil and avocado dressing. Mix and enjoy!

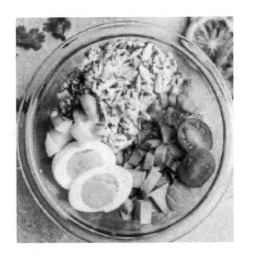

Nutritions:

Calories: 1093 kcal
Sugar: 17 g
Fat: 81 g

Protein: 68 g
Carbohydrates: 34 g

152. KETO CHICKEN SALAD

INGREDIENTS

- 2 cups cooked chicken, shredded
- 2 boiled eggs, chopped
- ¼ cup pecans, chopped
- ¼ cup dill pickles, chopped
- ½ cup mayonnaise
- ¼ cup minced yellow onion
- 1 tsp. yellow mustard
- 1 tsp. white distilled vinegar
- 1 tsp. fresh dill
- Salt and pepper to taste

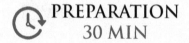 **PREPARATION** 30 MIN 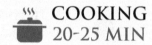 **COOKING** 20-25 MIN 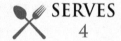 **SERVES** 4

DIRECTIONS

1. Except for the chicken, add everything together in a mixing bowl and stir together until thoroughly combined.
2. Add the chicken and stir well, making sure that the whole chicken is well coated.
3. Add salt and pepper to taste.
4. Chill in the fridge for one hour before serving. You can keep it stored in the fridge for 3 to 5 days.

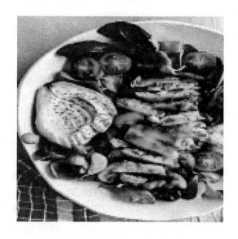

Nutritions:

Calories: 394 kcal
Saturated fat: 33 g
Trans fat: 6 g

Cholesterol: 25 g
Carbohydrates: 3 g
Sugar: 1 g

Protein: 21 g

153. TUNA FISH SALAD – QUICK AND EASY!

INGREDIENTS

- 10 kalamata olives, pitted 1 small zucchini sliced lengthwise
- ½ diced avocado 2 cups mixed greens 1 large diced tomato
- 1 sliced green onion
- 1 can chunk light tuna in water, drained ¼ cup fresh parsley, chopped
- ½ cup fresh mint, chopped
- 1 tbsp. extra virgin olive oil
- 1 tbsp. balsamic vinegar
- ¼ tsp. fine sea salt
- ¾ tsp. black pepper, cracked

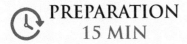 **PREPARATION** 15 MIN   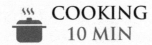 **COOKING** 10 MIN   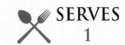 **SERVES** 1

DIRECTIONS

1. Grill the zucchini slices on both sides for a few minutes or as desired. Once cooked, cut it into bite-size pieces.
2. Grab a large bowl and just put all the ingredients together in the container, mixing them together until the liquid Ingredients are evenly distributed.
3. Serve while still fresh. This salad would taste best if eaten immediately so try not to have any leftovers.

Nutritions:

Calories: 563 kcal
Total fat: 30.9 g
Carbohydrates: 37.5 g

Dietary fiber: 15.7 g
Protein: 41.8 g

154. POTLUCK LAMB SALAD

INGREDIENTS

- 2 tbsp. olive oil, divided
- 12 oz. grass-fed lamb leg steaks, trimmed
- Salt and ground black pepper,
- 6½ oz. halloumi cheese, cut into thick slices
- 2 jarred roasted red bell peppers, sliced thinly
- 2 cucumbers, cut into thin ribbons
- 3 C. fresh baby spinach
- 2 tbsp. balsamic vinegar

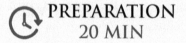 **PREPARATION** 20 MIN

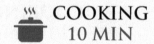 **COOKING** 10 MIN

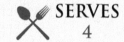 **SERVES** 4

DIRECTIONS

1. In a skillet, heat 1 tbsp. of the oil over medium-high heat and cook the lamb steaks for about 4-5 minutes per side or until desired doneness.
2. Transfer the lamb steaks onto a cutting board for about 5 minutes.
3. Then cut the lamb steaks into thin slices.
4. In the same skillet, add halloumi and cook for about 1-2 minutes per side or until golden.
5. In a salad bowl, add the lamb, haloumi, bell pepper, cucumber, salad leaves, vinegar and remaining oil and toss to combine.
6. Serve immediately.

Nutritions:

Calories: 420 kcal
Carbohydrates: 8 g
Protein: 35.4 g

Fat: 27.2 g
Sugar: 4 g
Sodium: 417 mg

Fiber: 1.3g

155. SPRING SUPPER SALAD

INGREDIENTS

- **For Salad:**
- 1 lb. fresh asparagus, cut into 1-inch pieces and trimmed
- ½ lb. smoked salmon, cut into bite-sized pieces
- 2 heads red leaf lettuce, torn   ¼ C. pecans, toasted and chopped

- **For Dressing:**
- ¼ C. olive oil
- 2 tbsp. fresh lemon juice
- 1 tsp. Dijon mustard
- Salt and ground black pepper

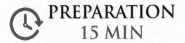 **PREPARATION**
15 MIN

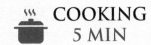 **COOKING**
5 MIN

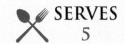 **SERVES**
5

DIRECTIONS

1. In a pan of boiling water, add the asparagus and cook for about 5 minutes.
2. Drain the asparagus well.
3. In a serving bowl, add the asparagus and remaining salad ingredients and mix.
4. In another bowl, add all the dressing ingredients and beat until well combined.
5. Place the dressing over salad and gently, toss to coat well.
6. Serve immediately.

Nutritions:

Calories: 223 kcal
Carbohydrates: 8.5 g
Protein: 11.7 g

Fat: 17.2 g
Sugar: 3.4 g
Sodium: 960 mg

Fiber: 3.5g

156. CHICKEN-OF-SEA SALAD

INGREDIENTS

- 2 (6-oz.) cans olive oil packed tuna, drained
- 2 (6-oz.) cans water packed tuna, drained
- ¾ C. mayonnaise
- 2 celery stalks, chopped
- ¼ of onion, chopped
- 1 tbsp. fresh lime juice
- 2 tbsp. mustard
- Freshly ground black pepper, to taste
- 6 C. fresh baby arugula

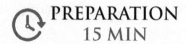 **PREPARATION**
15 MIN

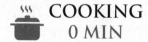 **COOKING**
0 MIN

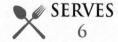 **SERVES**
6

DIRECTIONS

1. Add all the ingredients except arugula into a bowl and gently stir to combine.
2. Divide arugula onto serving plates and top with tuna mixture.
3. Serve immediately.

Nutritions:

Calories: 325 kcal
Carbohydrates: 2.7 g
Protein: 27.4 g

Fat: 22.2 g
Sugar: 0.9 g
Sodium: 389 mg

Fiber: 1.1 g

157. BACON AVOCADO SALAD

INGREDIENTS

- 2 hard-boiled eggs, chopped
- 2 cups spinach
- 2 large avocados, 1 chopped and 1 sliced
- 2 small lettuce heads, chopped
- 1 spring onion, sliced
- 4 cooked bacon slices, crumbled

VINAIGRETTE:
- 3 tablespoons olive oil
- 1 teaspoon Dijon mustard
- 1 tablespoon apple cider vinegar

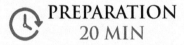 **PREPARATION**
20 MIN

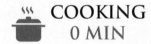 **COOKING**
0 MIN

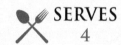 **SERVES**
4

DIRECTIONS

1. In a large bowl, mix together the eggs, spinach, avocados, lettuce, and onion.
2. In a separate bowl, add the olive oil, mustard, and apple cider vinegar. Mix well.
3. Pour the vinaigrette into the large bowl and toss well.
4. Serve topped with bacon slices and sliced avocado.

TIP: To add more flavors to this meal, serve with a sprinkle of Parmesan cheese.

Nutritions:

Calories: 342.5 kcal

Net Carbs: 3.5 g

Fat: 33.3 g

Protein: 7.2 g

158. CAULIFLOWER, SHRIMP AND CUCUMBER SALAD

INGREDIENTS

- ¼ cup olive oil
- 1 pound (454 g) medium shrimp
- 1 cauliflower head, florets only
- 2 cucumber, peeled and chopped

DRESSING:
- 1 tablespoon olive oil
- ¼ cup lemon juice
- 2 tablespoons lemon zest
- 3 tablespoons dill, chopped
- Salt and pepper, to taste

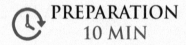 **PREPARATION** 10 MIN

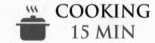 **COOKING** 15 MIN

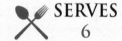 **SERVES** 6

DIRECTIONS

1. In a skillet over medium heat, heat the olive oil until sizzling hot. Add the shrimp and cook for 8 minutes, stirring occasionally, or until the flesh is totally pink and opaque.
2. Meanwhile, in a microwave-safe bowl, add the cauliflower florets and microwave for about 5 minutes until tender.
3. Remove the shrimp from the heat to a large bowl. Add the cauliflower and cucumber to the shrimp in the bowl. Set aside.
4. Make the dressing: Mix together the olive oil, lemon juice, lemon zest, dill, salt, and pepper in a third bowl. Pour the dressing into the bowl of shrimp mixture. Toss well until the shrimp and vegetables are coated thoroughly.
5. Serve immediately or refrigerate for 1 hour before serving.

TIP: The shrimp can be cooked ahead of time, cooled completely, and cover with plastic wrap in the refrigerator until you make the salad.

Nutritions:

Calories: 236.9 kcal
Fat: 17.3 g
Protein: 15.2 g

Net Carbs: 5.1 g

159. SEARED SQUID SALAD WITH RED CHILI DRESSING

INGREDIENTS

- 4 medium squid tubes, cut into rings
- 1 tablespoon chopped cilantro, for garnish

SALAD:
- 1 cup arugula
- 2 medium cucumbers, halved and cut into strips
- ½ red onion, finely sliced
- ½ cup mint leaves
- ½ cup cilantro leaves, reserve the stems
- Salt and black pepper, to taste

- 2 tablespoons olive oil, divided

DRESSING:
- 1 red chili, roughly chopped
- 1 clove garlic
- 1 teaspoon Swerve
- 2 limes, juiced
- 1 teaspoon fish sauce

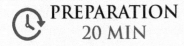 **PREPARATION** 20 MIN

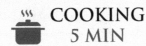 **COOKING** 5 MIN

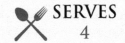 **SERVES** 4

DIRECTIONS

1. Make the salad: Mix together the arugula, cucumber strips, red onion, mint leaves, and coriander leaves in a salad bowl. Add the salt, pepper, and 1 tablespoon olive oil. Toss to combine well and set aside.
2. Make the dressing: Lightly pound the red chili, garlic clove, and Swerve in a clay mortar with a wooden pestle until it forms a coarse paste. Mix in the lime juice and fish sauce. Set aside.
3. Warm the residual olive oil in a skillet over high heat. Add the squid and sear for about 5 minutes until lightly browned.
4. Transfer the squid to the salad bowl and top with the dressing. Stir well. Serve garnished with the cilantro.

TIP: For a unique twist, you can make this salad with beef besides squid.

Nutritions:

Calories: 332.5 kcal
Fat: 24.5 g
Protein: 23.5 g

Net Carbs: 4.5 g

160. CAULIFLOWER AND CASHEW NUT SALAD

INGREDIENTS

- 1 head cauliflower, cut into florets
- ½ cup black olives, pitted and chopped
- 1 cup roasted bell peppers, chopped
- 1 red onion, sliced
- ½ cup cashew nuts
- Chopped celery leaves, for garnish

DRESSING:
- ¼ cup extra-virgin olive oil
- 1 teaspoon yellow mustard
- 1 tablespoon wine vinegar
- Salt and black pepper, to taste

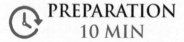 **PREPARATION** 10 MIN   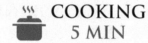 **COOKING** 5 MIN   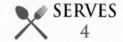 **SERVES** 4

DIRECTIONS

1. Add the cauliflower into a pot of boiling salted water. Allow to boil for 4 to 5 minutes until fork-tender but still crisp.
2. Remove from the heat and drain on paper towels, then transfer the cauliflower to a bowl.
3. Add the olives, bell pepper, and red onion. Stir well.
4. Mix together the olive oil, mustard, vinegar, salt, and pepper. Pour the dressing over the veggies and toss to combine. On a separate bowl.
5. Serve topped with cashew nuts and celery leaves.

TIP: Blanching the cauliflower can give it a desired and uniform texture.

Nutritions:

Calories: 196.7 kcal   Net Carbs: 6.2 g
Fat: 16.3 g
Protein: 6.3 g

161. SALMON AND LETTUCE SALAD

INGREDIENTS

- 1 tablespoon extra-virgin olive oil
- 2 slices smoked salmon, chopped
- 3 tablespoons mayonnaise
- 1 tablespoon lime juice
- Sea salt, to taste
- 1 cup romaine lettuce, shredded
- 1 teaspoon onion flakes
- ½ avocado, sliced

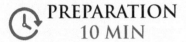 **PREPARATION**
10 MIN

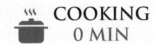 **COOKING**
0 MIN

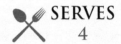 **SERVES**
4

DIRECTIONS

1. In a bowl, stir together the olive oil, salmon, mayo, lime juice, and salt. Stir well until the salmon is coated fully.
2. Divide evenly the romaine lettuce and onion flakes among four serving plates. Spread the salmon mixture over the lettuce, then serve topped with avocado slices.

TIP: The taste of avocado slices will be much stronger if you refrigerate the salad for 30 minutes before serving.

Nutritions:

Calories: 227.1 kcal
Fat: 20.3 g
Protein: 8.8 g

Net Carbs: 2.3 g

162. PRAWNS SALAD WITH MIXED LETTUCE GREENS

INGREDIENTS

- ½ pound (227 g) prawns, peeled and deveined
- Salt and chili pepper, to taste
- 1 tablespoon olive oil
- 2 cups mixed lettuce greens

DRESSING:
- ½ teaspoon Dijon mustard
- ¼ cup aioli
- 1 tablespoon lemon juice

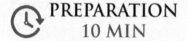 **PREPARATION** 10 MIN

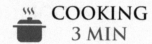 **COOKING** 3 MIN

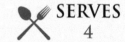 **SERVES** 4

DIRECTIONS

1. In a bowl, add the prawns, salt, and chili pepper. Toss well.
2. Warm the olive oil over medium heat. Add the seasoned prawns and fry for about 6 to 8 minutes, stirring occasionally, or until the prawns are opaque.
3. Remove from the heat and set the prawns aside on a platter.
4. Make the dressing: In a small bowl, mix together the mustard, aioli, and lemon juice until creamy and smooth.
5. Make the salad: In a separate bowl, add the mixed lettuce greens. Pour the dressing over the greens and toss to combine.
6. Divide the salad among four servings and serve it alongside the prawns.

TIP: The prawns can be done ahead, cooled completely, and cover with plastic wrap in the refrigerator until you serve the salad.

Nutritions:

Calories: 226.9 kcal
Fat: 21.3 g
Protein: 6.9 g

Net Carbs: 1.9 g

163. POACHED EGG SALAD WITH LETTUCE AND OLIVES

INGREDIENTS

- 4 eggs
- 1 head romaine lettuce, torn into pieces
- ¼ stalk celery, minced
- ¼ cup mayonnaise
- ½ tablespoon mustard
- ½ teaspoon low-carb sriracha sauce
- ¼ teaspoon fresh lime juice
- Salt and black pepper, to taste
- ¼ cup chopped scallions, for garnish
- Sliced black olives, for garnish

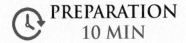 **PREPARATION** 10 MIN   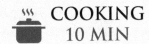 **COOKING** 10 MIN   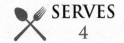 **SERVES** 4

DIRECTIONS

1. Put the eggs into a pot of salted water over medium heat, then bring to a boil for about 8 minutes.
2. Using a slotted spoon, remove the eggs one at a time from the hot water. Let them cool under running cold water in the sink. When cooled, peel the eggs and slice into bite-sized pieces, then transfer to a large bowl.
3. Make the salad: Add the romaine lettuce, stalk celery, mayo, mustard, sriracha sauce, lime juice, salt, and pepper to the bowl of egg pieces. Toss to combine well.
4. Divide the salad among four servings. Serve garnished with scallions and sliced black olives.

TIP: You can store the salad in a sealed airtight container in the fridge for up to 2 to 3 days. It is not recommended to freeze.

Nutritions:

Calories: 291.8 kcal
Fat: 21.8 g
Protein: 17.7 g

Net Carbs: 6.2 g

164. BEEF SALAD WITH VEGETABLES

INGREDIENTS

MEATBALLS:
- 1 pound (454 g) ground beef
- ¼ cup pork rinds, crushed
- 1 egg, whisked
- 1 onion, grated
- 1 tablespoon fresh parsley, chopped
- ½ teaspoon dried oregano
- 1 garlic clove, minced
- Salt and black pepper, to taste
- 2 tablespoons olive oil, divided

SALAD:
- 1 cup chopped arugula
- 1 cucumber, sliced
- 1 cup cherry tomatoes, halved
- 1½ tablespoons lemon juice
- Salt and pepper, to taste

DRESSING:
- 2 tablespoons almond milk
- 1 cup plain Greek yogurt
- 1 tablespoon fresh mint, chopped

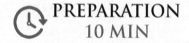 **PREPARATION** 10 MIN

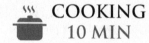 **COOKING** 10 MIN

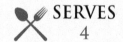 **SERVES** 4

DIRECTIONS

1. Stir together the beef, pork rinds, whisked egg, onion, parsley, oregano, garlic, salt, and pepper in a large bowl until completely mixed.
2. Make the meatballs: On a lightly floured surface, using a cookie scoop to scoop out equal-sized amounts of the beef mixture and form into meatballs with your palm.
3. Heat 1 tablespoon olive oil in a large skillet over medium heat, fry the meatballs for about 4 minutes on each side until cooked through.
4. Remove from the heat and set aside on a plate to cool.
5. In a salad bowl, mix together the arugula, cucumber, cherry tomatoes, 1 tablespoon olive oil, and lemon juice. Season with salt and pepper.
6. Make the dressing: In a third bowl, whisk the almond milk, yogurt, and mint until well blended. Pour the mixture over the salad. Serve topped with the meatballs.
7. TIP: If you don't have a large skillet that fits all the meatballs, you can cook them in batches.

Nutritions:

Calories: 487.2 kcal
Fat: 31.6 g
Protein: 42.2 g

Net Carbs: 8.5 g

165. NIÇOISE SALAD

INGREDIENTS

- ¾ cup MCT oil
- ½ cup lemon juice
- 1 teaspoon Dijon mustard
- 1 tablespoon fresh thyme leaves, minced
- 1 medium shallot, minced
- 2 teaspoons fresh oregano leaves, minced
- 2 tablespoons fresh basil leaves, minced
- Celtic sea salt and freshly ground black pepper, to taste

SALAD:
- 2 tablespoons butter
- 1 tablespoon olive oil

- 2 (8-ounce / 227-g) tuna steaks
- 2 heads of red leaf lettuce, wash and tear into bite-sized pieces
- ounces (227 g) green beans, stem ends trimmed and each bean halved crosswise
- 6 hard-boiled eggs, peeled and quartered
- 1 can anchovies, or more as needed
- 1 avocado, peeled and sliced into chunks
- 3 small tomatoes, sliced
- ¼ cup olives

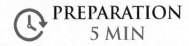 **PREPARATION** 5 MIN

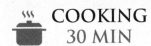 **COOKING** 30 MIN

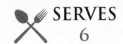 **SERVES** 6

DIRECTIONS

1. Melt butter and put olive oil in\ a nonstick skillet over medium-high heat. Place the tuna steaks in the skillet, and sear for 3 minutes or until opaque, flipping once. Set aside.
2. Make the dressing: Combine all the ingredients for the dressing in a bowl.
3. Make six niçoise salads: Dunk the lettuce and tuna steaks in the dressing bowl to coat well, then arrange the tuna in the middle of the lettuce. Set aside.
4. Blanch the green beans in a pot of boiling salted water for 3 to 5 minutes or until soft but still crisp. Drain and dry

with paper towels.
5. Dunk the green beans in the dressing bowl to coat well. Arrange them around the tuna steaks on the lettuce.
6. Top the tuna and green beans with hard-boiled eggs, anchovies, avocado chunks, tomatoes, and olives. Sprinkle 2 tablespoons dressing over each egg, then serve.

TIP: To make this a complete meal, you can top it with grilled rib eye steak or serve it with salmon soup and roasted duck.

Nutritions:

Calories: 502 kcal
Total Fat: 42.2 g
Carbs: 8.8 g

Protein: 23.6 g

166. SHRIMP, TOMATO, AND AVOCADO SALAD

INGREDIENTS

- 1 pound (454 g) shrimp, shelled and deveined
- 2 tomatoes, cubed
- 2 avocados, peeled and cubed
- A handful of fresh cilantro, chopped
- 4 green onions, minced
- Juice of 1 lime or lemon
- 1 tablespoon macadamia nut or avocado oil
- Celtic sea salt and ground black pepper,

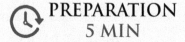 **PREPARATION** 5 MIN

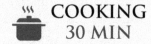 **COOKING** 30 MIN

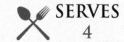 **SERVES** 4

DIRECTIONS

1. Combine the shrimp, tomatoes, avocados, cilantro, and onions in a large bowl.
2. Squeeze the lemon juice over the vegetables in the large bowl, then drizzle with avocado oil and sprinkle the salt and black pepper to season. Toss to combine well.
3. You can cover the salad, and refrigerate to chill for 45 minutes or serve immediately.

TIP: To make this a complete meal, you can top it with grilled rib eye steak or serve it with chicken soup and roasted turkey.

Nutritions:

Calories: 382 kcal
Total Fat: 27.2 g
Carbs: 5.8 g

Protein: 28.1 g

167. SIMPLE SAUTÉED ASPARAGUS SPEARS WITH WALNUTS

INGREDIENTS

- 1½ tablespoons olive oil
- ¾ pound (340 g) asparagus spears, woody ends trimmed
- Sea salt and ground pepper
- ¼ cup walnuts, chopped

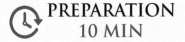 **PREPARATION**
10 MIN

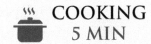 **COOKING**
5 MIN

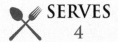 **SERVES**
4

DIRECTIONS

1. In a skillet over medium-high heat, heat the olive oil.
2. Add the asparagus and sauté for about 5 minutes until fork-tender, stirring occasionally.
3. Season with salt and pepper, then transfer to a large bowl.
4. Serve topped with chopped walnuts.

TIP: Blanching the asparagus can give it a smoother texture and an irresistible flavor.

Nutritions:

Calories: 131.9 kcal
Fat: 12.3 g
Protein: 3.2 g

Net Carbs: 2.1 g
Fiber: 2 g

168. CAULIFLOWER MASH

INGREDIENTS

- 1 head cauliflower, chopped roughly
- ¼ cup heavy whipping cream
- ½ cup shredded Cheddar cheese
- 2 tablespoons butter, at room temperature
- Sea salt and ground black pepper

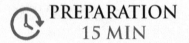 **PREPARATION** 15 MIN 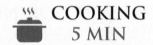 **COOKING** 5 MIN 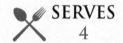 **SERVES** 4

DIRECTIONS

1. Fill a large saucepan three-quarters full with water and bring the water to a boil over high heat
2. Blanch the cauliflower in the boiling water for about 4 to 5 minutes, until it starts to soften.
3. Remove from the heat and drain on a paper towel.
4. Put the cauliflower in a food processor, along with the heavy cream, cheese, and butter. Process until it's creamy and fluffy. Sprinkle with salt and pepper.
5. Divide the cauliflower mixture among four serving bowls, and serve.

TIP: The cauliflower mash perfectly goes well with baked coconut chicken.

Nutritions:

Calories: 193.7 kcal
Fat: 15.3 g
Protein: 8.2 g

Net Carbs: 5.8 g
Fiber: 2 g

169. TENDER ZUCCHINI WITH CHEESE

INGREDIENTS

- 2 tablespoons butter
- 4 zucchinis, cut into ¼-inch-thick rounds
- ½ cup freshly grated Parmesan cheese
- Freshly ground black pepper, to taste

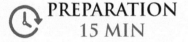 **PREPARATION**
15 MIN

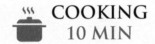 **COOKING**
10 MIN

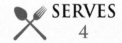 **SERVES**
4

DIRECTIONS

1. Melt the butter in a large frying pan over medium-high heat.
2. Sauté the zucchini in the melted butter for about 5 minutes, stirring frequently, or until the zucchini is tender but still crisp.
3. Scatter the grated Parmesan cheese over the zucchini. Cook for 5 minutes more until the cheese melts. Season as desired with salt and pepper.
4. Remove from the heat and serve on plates.

TIP: To add more flavors to this meal, garnish it with fresh basil or a handful of chopped chives.

Nutritions:

Calories: 95.9 kcal
Fat: 8.3 g
Protein: 4.2 g

Net Carbs: 1.1 g
Fiber: 0 g

170. TOFU SESAME SKEWERS WITH WARM KALE SALAD

INGREDIENTS

- oz Firm tofu
- tsp. sesame oil
- 1 lemon, juiced
- tbsp. sugar-free soy sauce
- 3 tsp. garlic powder
- tbsp. coconut flour
- 1/2 cup sesame seeds

Warm Kale Salad:
- Cups chopped kale
- 2 tsp. + 2 tsp. olive oil
- 1 white onion, thinly sliced
- 3 cloves garlic, minced
- 1 cup sliced white mushrooms
- 1 tsp. chopped rosemary
- Salt and black pepper to season
- 1 tbsp. balsamic vinegar

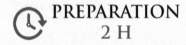 **PREPARATION** 2 H

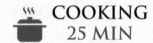 **COOKING** 25 MIN

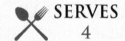 **SERVES** 4

DIRECTIONS

1. In a bowl, mix sesame oil, lemon juice, soy sauce, garlic powder, and coconut flour.
2. Wrap the tofu in a paper towel, squeeze out as much liquid from it, and cut it into strips.
3. Stick on the skewers, height-wise.
4. Place onto a plate, pour the soy sauce mixture over, and turn in the sauce to be adequately coated.
5. Heat the griddle pan over high heat.
6. Pour the sesame seeds on a plate and roll the tofu skewers in the seeds for a generous coat.
7. Grill the tofu in the griddle pan to be golden brown on both sides, about 12 minutes.

8. Heat 2 tablespoons of olive oil in a skillet over medium heat and sauté onion to begin browning for 10 minutes with continuous stirring.
9. Add the remaining olive oil and mushrooms.
10. Continue cooking for 10 minutes. Add garlic, rosemary, salt, pepper, and balsamic vinegar.
11. Cook for 1 minute.
12. Put the kale in a salad bowl; when the onion mixture is ready, pour it on the kale and toss well.
13. Serve the tofu skewers with the warm kale salad and a peanut butter dipping sauce.

Nutritions:

Calories: 276 kcal
Fat: 11.9 g
Fiber: 9.4 g

Carbohydrates: 21 g
Protein: 10.3 g

171. EGGPLANT PIZZA WITH TOFU

INGREDIENTS

- eggplants, sliced
- 1/3 cup butter, melted
- 2 garlic cloves, minced
- 1 red onion
- oz tofu, chopped
- oz tomato sauce
- Salt and black pepper to taste
- 1/2 tsp. cinnamon powder
- 1 cup Parmesan cheese, shredded
- 1/4 cup dried oregano

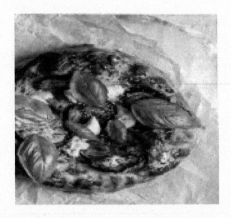

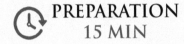 **PREPARATION** 15 MIN

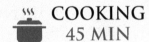 **COOKING** 45 MIN

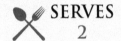 **SERVES** 2

DIRECTIONS

1. Let the oven heat to 400F. Lay the eggplant slices on a baking sheet and brush with some butter. Bake in the oven until lightly browned, about 20 minutes.
2. Heat the remaining butter in a skillet; sauté garlic and onion until fragrant and soft, about 3 minutes.
3. Stir in the tofu and cook for 3 minutes. Add the tomato sauce, salt and black pepper. Simmer for 10 minutes.
4. Sprinkle with the Parmesan cheese and oregano. Bake for 10 minutes.

Nutritions:

Calories: 321 kcal
Fat: 11.3 g
Fiber: 8.4 g

Carbohydrates: 4.3 g
Protein: 10.1 g

172. BRUSSEL SPROUTS WITH SPICED HALLOUMI

INGREDIENTS

- oz halloumi cheese, sliced
- 1 tbsp. coconut oil
- 1/2 cup unsweetened coconut, shredded
- 1 tsp. chili powder
- 1/2 tsp. onion powder
- 1/2 pound Brussels sprouts, shredded
- oz butter
- Salt and black pepper to taste
- Lemon wedges for serving

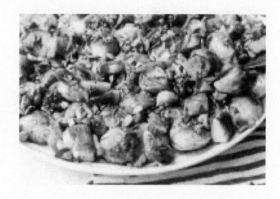

PREPARATION
20 MIN

COOKING
30 MIN

SERVES
2

DIRECTIONS

1. In a bowl, mix the shredded coconut, chili powder, salt, coconut oil, and onion powder.
2. Then, toss the halloumi slices in the spice mixture.
3. The grill pan must be heated then cook the coated halloumi cheese for 2-3 minutes.
4. Transfer to a plate to keep warm.
5. The half butter must be melted in a pan, add, and sauté the Brussels sprouts until slightly caramelized.
6. Then, season with salt and black pepper.
7. Dish the Brussels sprouts into serving plates with the halloumi cheese and lemon wedges.
8. Melt left butter and drizzle over the Brussels sprouts and halloumi cheese. Serve.

Nutritions:

Calories: 276 kcal
Fat: 9.5 g
Fiber: 9.1 g

Carbohydrates: 4.1 g
Protein: 5.4 g

173. CHEESY STUFFED PEPPERS

INGREDIENTS

- tbsp. olive oil
- red bell peppers, halved and seeded
- 1 cup ricotta cheese
- 1/2 cup gorgonzola cheese, crumbled
- 2 cloves garlic, minced
- 1 1/2 cups tomatoes, chopped
- 1 tsp. dried basil
- Salt and black pepper, to taste
- 1/2 tsp. oregano

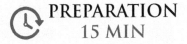 **PREPARATION** 15 MIN

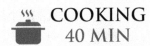 **COOKING** 40 MIN

 **SERVES** 4

DIRECTIONS

1. Let the oven heat up to 350F.
2. In a bowl, mix garlic, tomatoes, gorgonzola, and ricotta cheeses.
3. Stuff the pepper halves and remove them to the baking dish. Season with oregano, salt, cayenne pepper, black pepper, and basil.
4. Baking Time: 40 minutes

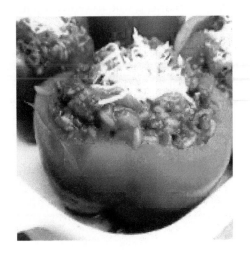

Nutritions:

Calories: 295 kcal
Fat: 12.4 g
Fiber: 10.1 g

Carbohydrates: 5.4 g
Protein: 13.2 g

174. VEGETABLE PATTIES

INGREDIENTS

- 1 tbsp. olive oil
- 1 onion, chopped
- 1 garlic clove, minced
- 1/2 head cauliflower, grated
- 1 carrot, shredded
- tbsp. coconut flour
- 1/2 cup Gruyere cheese, shredded
- 1/2 cup Parmesan cheese, grated
- 2 eggs, beaten
- 1/2 tsp. dried rosemary
- Salt and black pepper, to taste

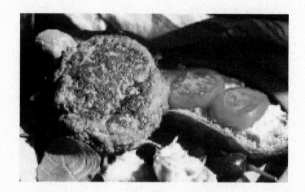

PREPARATION 15 MIN

COOKING 20 MIN

SERVES 4

DIRECTIONS

1. Cook onion and garlic in warm olive oil over medium heat, until soft, for about 3 minutes.
2. Stir in grated cauliflower and carrot and cook for a minute; allow cooling and set aside.
3. To the cooled vegetables, add the rest of the ingredients, form balls from the mixture, then press each ball to form a burger patty.
4. Set oven to 400 F and bake the burgers for 20 minutes.
5. Flip and bake for another 10 minutes or until the top becomes golden brown.

Nutritions:

Calories: 315 kcal
Fat: 12.1 g
Fiber: 8.6 g

Carbohydrates: 3.3 g
Protein: 5.8 g

175. VEGAN SANDWICH WITH TOFU & LETTUCE SLAW

INGREDIENTS

- 1/4 pound firm tofu, sliced
- low carb buns
- 1 tbsp. olive oil
- Marinade
- 2 tbsp. olive oil
- Salt and black pepper to taste
- 1 tsp. allspice
- 1/2 tbsp. xylitol
- 1 tsp. thyme, chopped
- 1 habanero pepper, seeded and minced
- 2 green onions, thinly sliced
- 1 garlic clove

- Lettuce slaw
- 1/2 small iceberg lettuce, shredded
- 1/2 carrot, grated
- 1/2 red onion, grated
- 2 tsp. liquid stevia
- 1 tbsp. lemon juice
- 2 tbsp. olive oil
- 1/2 tsp. Dijon mustard
- Salt and black pepper to taste

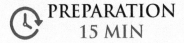 **PREPARATION** 15 MIN

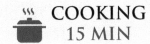 **COOKING** 15 MIN

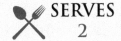 **SERVES** 2

DIRECTIONS

1. Put the tofu slices in a bowl.
2. Blend the marinade ingredients for a minute.
3. Cover the tofu with this mixture and place in the fridge to marinate for 1 hour.
4. In a container, combine the lemon juice, stevia, olive oil, Dijon mustard, salt, and pepper.
5. Stir in the lettuce, carrot, and onion; set aside.
6. Heat oil, cook the tofu on both sides for 6 minutes in total.
7. Remove to a plate.
8. In the buns, add the tofu and top with the slaw. Close the buns and serve.

Nutritions:

Calories: 315 kcal
Fat: 10.4 g
Fiber: 15.1 g

Carbohydrates: 9.4 g
Protein: 8.4 g

176. PIZZA BIANCA

INGREDIENTS

- tbsp. olive oil
- eggs
- 2 tbsp. water
- 1 jalapeño pepper, diced
- 1/4 cup mozzarella cheese, shredded
- 2 chives, chopped
- 2 cups egg Alfredo sauce
- 1/2 tsp. oregano
- 1/2 cup mushrooms, sliced

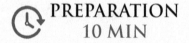 **PREPARATION** 10 MIN   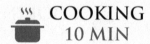 **COOKING** 10 MIN   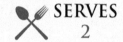 **SERVES** 2

DIRECTIONS

1. Preheat oven to 360 F.
2. In a bowl, whisk eggs, water, and oregano. Heat the olive oil in a large skillet.
3. The egg mixture must be poured in then let it cook until set, flipping once.
4. Remove and spread the Alfredo sauce and jalapeño pepper all over.
5. Top with mozzarella cheese, mushrooms and chives. Let it bake for 10 minutes

Nutritions:

Calories: 314 kcal
Fat: 15.6 g
Fiber: 10.3 g

Carbohydrates: 5.9 g
Protein: 10.4 g

177. GREEK VEGGIE BRIAM

INGREDIENTS

- 1/3 cup good-quality olive oil, divided
- 1 onion, thinly sliced
- 1 tablespoon minced garlic
- 3/4 small eggplant, diced
- zucchinis, diced
- 2 cups chopped cauliflower
- 1 red bell pepper, diced
- 2 cups diced tomatoes
- 2 tablespoons chopped fresh parsley
- 2 tablespoons chopped fresh oregano
- Sea salt, for seasoning
- Freshly ground black pepper, for seasoning
- 11/2 cups crumbled feta cheese
- 1/4 cup pumpkin seeds

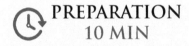 **PREPARATION** 10 MIN

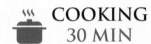 **COOKING** 30 MIN

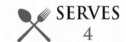 **SERVES** 4

DIRECTIONS

1. Preheat the oven. Set the oven to broil and lightly grease a 9-by-13-inch casserole dish with olive oil.
2. Sauté the aromatics in a medium stockpot over medium heat, warm 3 tablespoons of the olive oil. Add the onion and garlic and sauté until they've softened about 3 minutes.
3. Sauté the vegetables. Stir in the eggplant, cook, stirring occasionally.
4. Add the zucchini, cauliflower, and red bell pepper and cook for 5 minutes.
5. Stir in the tomatoes, parsley, and oregano and cook, stirring it from time to time, until the vegetables are tender, about 10 minutes. Season it with salt and pepper.
6. Broil. Put vegetable mix in the casserole dish and top with the crumbled feta. Broil until the cheese is melted.
7. Serve. Divide the casserole between four plates and top it with the pumpkin seeds. Drizzle with the remaining olive oil.

Nutritions:

Calories: 341 kcal
Fat: 5.1 g
Fiber: 11 g

Carbohydrates: 1.2 g
Protein: 1.4 g

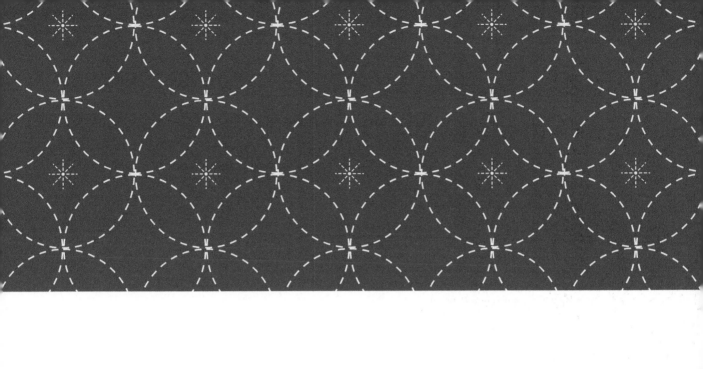

CHAPTER 12
SOUPS

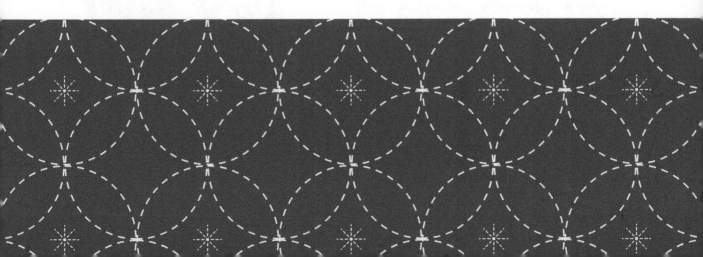

178. KETO SHIRATAKI SOUP

INGREDIENTS

- Boneless - skinless chicken thighs (2)
- Chicken stock (3 cups)
- Minced ginger (1 tsp.)
- Cardamom (.25 tsp.)
- Minced garlic (1 clove)
- Mushrooms (.5 cup)
- Optional: chili sauce (1 tsp.)
- Chopped cilantro (1 pinch)
- Thinly sliced chili pepper (1)

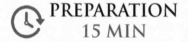 **PREPARATION**
15 MIN

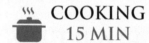 **COOKING**
15 MIN

 **SERVES**
2

DIRECTIONS

1. Warm up the stock on the stovetop using the med-high heat setting. Toss in the ginger, garlic, mushrooms, and cardamom. Simmer for about 10 minutes.
2. Fold in the chicken and cook until done or about 5 minutes.
3. Prepare two soup bowls and add the sliced chili pepper to each dish. Serve the soup and garnish with some cilantro.
4. Adjust spices to your liking.

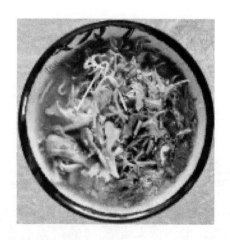

Nutritions:

Calories: 130 kcal
Protein: 29.4 g
Fat: 12 g

Net Carbohydrates: 1.5 g

179. KETO SLOW-COOKED BEEF STEW

INGREDIENTS

- Beef broth (1 cup)
- Organic chili-ready diced tomatoes (2 cans - 14.5 oz. Each)
- Hot sauce (2 tsp.)
- Stew beef (5 lb.)
- Prepackaged chili mix (1 tbsp.)
- Worcestershire sauce (1 tbsp.)
- Salt (to taste)

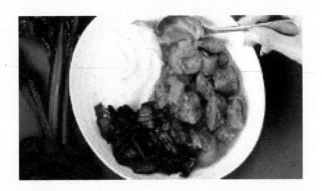

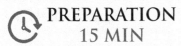 **PREPARATION** 15 MIN

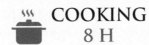 **COOKING** 8 H

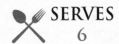 **SERVES** 6

DIRECTIONS

1. Prepare the slow cooker using the high-temperature setting.
2. Toss each of the fixings into the pot.
3. Set the timer for six hours. Break the meat apart and continue cooking for another two hours. Add a pinch of salt and serve.

Nutritions:

Calories: 222 kcal
Protein: 27 g
Fat Content: 7 g

Net Carbohydrates: 9 g

180. KETO-VEGAN POMODORO SOUP - INSTANT POT

INGREDIENTS

- Coconut cream (1 cup)
- Veggie broth (29 oz.)
- Tomatoes (3 lb.)
- Diced onion (1)
- Vegan butter (3 tbsp.)

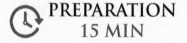 **PREPARATION**
15 MIN

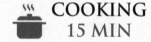 **COOKING**
15 MIN

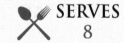 **SERVES**
8

DIRECTIONS

1. Warm the instant pot using the sauté function. Once it's hot, add the butter to melt and toss in the onions. Sauté for three to five minutes.
2. Mix in the tomatoes and simmer for another two minutes. Secure the lid and set the soup function for six minutes.
3. Press the cancel button and wait for about four to five minutes before you quick-pressure release. Stir in coconut cream to sauté for one minute.
4. Puree the soup using a hand mixer before serving.

Nutritions:

Calories: 300 kcal
Protein: 11 g
Fat Content: 18 g

Net Carbohydrates: 6.5 g

181. KETO BROCCOLI CURRY SOUP

INGREDIENTS

- Onion (1)
- Curry (1 tbsp.)
- Coconut oil (2 tbsp.)
- Vegetable stock (1 liter)
- Salt and black pepper (to taste)
- Coconut cream (1 cup)
- Cheese substitute - your choice of keto-friendly (75 g grated)
- Broccoli (1 lb.)

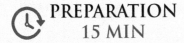 **PREPARATION** 15 MIN   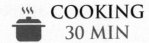 **COOKING** 30 MIN   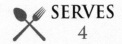 **SERVES** 4

DIRECTIONS

1. Prepare a skillet with coconut oil on the stovetop using the med-high temperature setting.
2. Chop the onion and sauté it for approximately six minutes.
3. Lower the temperature to medium and add in the broth until it begins to simmer.
4. Mix in the broccoli and seasonings before adding curry. Simmer it for 20 minutes.
5. Pour it into a blender before mixing in a keto-friendly cheese substitute.
6. Blend well.

Nutritions:

Calories: 375 kcal
Protein: 17 g
Fat Content: 20 g

Net Carbohydrates: 5 g

182. WINTER COMFORT STEW

INGREDIENTS

- 2 tbsp. Olive oil
- 1 small yellow onion, chopped
- 2 garlic cloves, chopped
- 2 lb. Grass-fed beef chuck, cut into 1-inch cubes
- 1 (14-oz.) Can sugar-free crushed tomatoes
- 2 tsp. Ground allspice
- 1½ tsp. Red pepper flakes
- ½ c. Homemade beef broth
- 6 oz. Green olives pitted
- oz. Fresh baby spinach
- 2 tbsp. Fresh lemon juice
- Salt and freshly ground black pepper, to taste
- ¼ c. Fresh cilantro, chopped

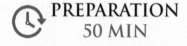 **PREPARATION**
50 MIN

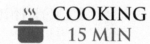 **COOKING**
15 MIN

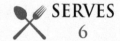 **SERVES**
6

DIRECTIONS

1. In a pan, heat the oil in a pan over high heat and sauté the onion and garlic for about 2-3 minutes.
2. Add the beef and cook for about 3-4 minutes or until browned, stirring frequently.
3. Add the tomatoes, spices and broth, and bring to a boil.
4. Reduce the heat to low and simmer, covered for about 30-40 minutes or until the desired doneness of the beef.
5. Stir in the olives and spinach and simmer for about 2-3 minutes.
6. Stir in the lemon juice, salt and black pepper and remove from the heat.
7. Serve hot with the garnishing of cilantro.

Nutritions:

Calories: 388 kcal
Carbohydrates: 8 g
Protein: 485 g

Fat: 17.7 g
Sugar: 2.6 g
Sodium: 473 mg

Fiber: 3.1 g

183. IDEAL COLD WEATHER STEW

INGREDIENTS

- 3 tbsp. Olive oil, divided
- oz. Fresh mushrooms, quartered
- 1¼ lb. Grass-fed beef chuck roast, trimmed and cubed into 1-inch size
- 2 tbsp. Tomato paste
- ½ tsp. Dried thyme
- 1 bay leaf
- 5 c. Homemade beef broth
- 6 oz. Celery root, peeled and cubed
- 4 oz. Yellow onions, chopped roughly
- 3 oz. Carrot, peeled and sliced
- 2 garlic cloves, sliced
- Salt and freshly ground black pepper, to taste

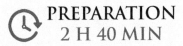 **PREPARATION** 2 H 40 MIN

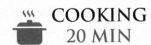 **COOKING** 20 MIN

 **SERVES** 6

DIRECTIONS

1. In a Dutch oven, heat 1 tbsp. Of the oil over medium heat and cook the mushrooms for about 2 minutes, without stirring.
2. Stir the mushroom and cook for about 2 minutes more.
3. With a slotted spoon, transfer the mushroom onto a plate.
4. In the same pan, heat the remaining oil over medium-high heat and sear the beef cubes for about 4-5 minutes.
5. Stir in the tomato paste, thyme and bay leaf, and cook for about 1 minute.
6. Stir in the broth and bring to a boil.
7. Reduce the heat to low and simmer, covered for about 1½ hours.
8. Stir in the mushrooms, celery, onion, carrot and garlic, and simmers for about 40-60 minutes.
9. Stir in the salt and black pepper and remove from the heat.
10. Serve hot.

Nutritions:

Calories: 447 kcal
Carbohydrates: 7.4 g
Protein: 30.8 g

Fat: 32.3 g
Sugar: 8 g
Sodium: 764 mg

Fiber: 1.9 g

184. WEEKEND DINNER STEW

INGREDIENTS

- 1½ lb. Grass-fed beef stew meat, trimmed and cubed into 1-inch size
- Salt and freshly ground black pepper, to taste
- 1 tbsp. Olive oil
- 1 c. Homemade tomato puree
- 4 c. Homemade beef broth
- 2 c. Zucchini, chopped
- 2 celery ribs, sliced
- ½ c. Carrots, peeled and sliced
- 2 garlic cloves, minced
- ½ tbsp. Dried thyme
- 1 tsp. Dried parsley
- 1 tsp. Dried rosemary
- 1 tbsp. Paprika
- 1 tsp. Onion powder
- 1 tsp. Garlic powder

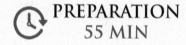 **PREPARATION** 55 MIN

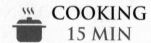 **COOKING** 15 MIN

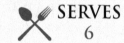 **SERVES** 6

DIRECTIONS

1. In a large bowl, add the beef cubes, salt and black pepper, and toss to coat well.
2. In a large pan, heat the oil over medium-high heat and cook the beef cubes for about 4-5 minutes or until browned.
3. Add the remaining ingredients and stir to combine.
4. Increase the heat to high and bring to a boil.
5. Reduce the heat to low and simmer, covered for about 40-50 minutes.
6. Stir in the salt and black pepper and remove from the heat.
7. Serve hot.

Nutritions:

Calories: 293 kcal
Carbohydrates: 8 g
Protein: 9.3 g

Fat: 10.7 g
Sugar: 4 g
Sodium: 223 mg

Fiber: 2.3 g

185. MEXICAN PORK STEW

INGREDIENTS

- 3 tbsp. Unsalted butter
- 2½ lb. Boneless pork ribs, cut into ¾-inch cubes
- 1 large yellow onion, chopped
- 4 garlic cloves, crushed
- 1½ c. Homemade chicken broth
- 2 (10-oz.) Cans sugar-free diced tomatoes
- 1 c. Canned roasted poblano chiles
- 2 tsp. Dried oregano
- 1 tsp. Ground cumin
- Salt, to taste
- ¼ c. Fresh cilantro, chopped
- 2 tbsp. Fresh lime juice

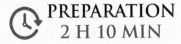 **PREPARATION** 2 H 10 MIN

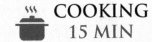 **COOKING** 15 MIN

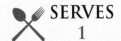 **SERVES** 1

DIRECTIONS

1. In a large pan, melt the butter over medium-high heat and cook the pork, onions and garlic for about 5 minutes or until browned.
2. Add the broth and scrape up the browned bits.
3. Add the tomatoes, poblano chiles, oregano, cumin, and salt and bring to a boil.
4. Reduce the heat to medium-low and simmer, covered for about 2 hours.
5. Stir in the fresh cilantro and lime juice and remove from heat.
6. Serve hot.

Nutritions:

Calories: 288 kcal
Carbohydrates: 8.8 g
Protein: 39.6 g

Fat: 10.1 g
Sugar: 4 g
Sodium: 283 mg

Fiber: 2.8 g

186. HUNGARIAN PORK STEW

INGREDIENTS

- 3 tbsp. olive oil
- 3½ lb. pork shoulder, cut into 4 portions
- 1 tbsp. butter
- 2 medium onions, chopped
- 16 oz. tomatoes, crushed
- 5 garlic cloves, crushed
- 2 Hungarian wax peppers, chopped
- 3 tbsp. Hungarian Sweet paprika
- 1 tbsp. smoked paprika
- 1 tsp. hot paprika
- ½ tsp. caraway seeds
- 1 bay leaf

- 1 C. homemade chicken broth
- 1 packet unflavored gelatin
- 2 tbsp. fresh lemon juice
- Pinch of xanthan gum
- Salt and freshly ground black pepper, to taste

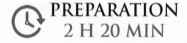 **PREPARATION** 2 H 20 MIN

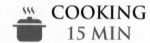 **COOKING** 15 MIN

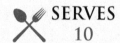 **SERVES** 10

DIRECTIONS

1. In a heavy-bottomed pan, heat 1 tbsp. Of oil over high heat and sear the pork for about 2-3 minutes or until browned.
2. Transfer the pork onto a plate and cut it into bite-sized pieces.
3. In the same pan, heat 1 tbsp. of oil and butter over medium-low heat and sauté the onions for about 5-6 minutes.
4. With a slotted spoon, transfer the onion into a bowl.
5. In the same pan, add the tomatoes and cook for about 3-4 minutes, without stirring.
6. Meanwhile, in a small frying pan, heat the remaining oil over low heat and sauté the garlic, wax peppers, all kinds of paprika and caraway seeds for about 20-30 seconds.
7. Remove from the heat and set aside.
8. In a small bowl, mix together the gelatin and broth.
9. In the large pan, add the cooked pork, garlic mixture, gelatin mixture and bay leaf and bring t0 a gentle boil.
10. Reduce the heat to low and simmer, covered for about 2 hours.
11. Stir in the xanthan gum and simmer for about 3-5 minutes.
12. Stir in the lemon juice, salt and black pepper and remove from the heat.
13. Serve hot.

Nutritions:

Calories: 529 kcal
Carbohydrates: 5.8 g
Protein: 38.9 g

Fat: 38.5 g
Sugar: 2.6 g
Sodium: 216 mg

Fiber: 2.1 g

187. YELLOW CHICKEN SOUP

INGREDIENTS

- 2½ tsp. ground turmeric
- 1½ tsp. ground cumin
- 1/8 tsp cayenne pepper
- 2 tbsp. butter, divided
- 1 small yellow onion, chopped
- 2 C. cauliflower, chopped
- 2 C. broccoli, chopped
- 4 C. homemade chicken broth
- 1½ C. water
- 1 tsp. fresh ginger root, grated
- 1 bay leaf
- 2 C. Swiss chard stemmed and chopped

- finely
- ½ C. unsweetened coconut milk
- 3 (4-oz.) grass-fed boneless, skinless chicken thighs, cut into bite-size pieces
- 2 tbsp. fresh lime juice

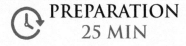 **PREPARATION** 25 MIN   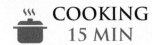 **COOKING** 15 MIN   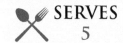 **SERVES** 5

DIRECTIONS

1. In a small bowl, mix together the turmeric, cumin and cayenne pepper and set aside.
2. Ina large pan, melt 1 tbsp. of the butter over medium heat and sauté the onion for about 3-4 minutes.
3. Add the cauliflower, broccoli and half of the spice mixture and cook for another 3-4 minutes.
4. Add the broth, water, ginger and bay leaf and bring to a boil.
5. Reduce the heat to low and simmer for about 8-10 minutes.
6. Stir in the Swiss chard and coconut milk and cook for about 1-2 minutes.
7. Meanwhile, in a large skillet, melt the remaining butter over medium heat and sear the chicken pieces for about 5 minutes.
8. Stir in the remaining spice mix and cook for about 5 minutes, stirring frequently.
9. Transfer the soup into serving bowls and top with the chicken pieces.
10. Drizzle with lime juice and serve.

Nutritions:

Calories: 258 kcal
Carbohydrates: 8.4 g
Protein: 18.4 g

Fat: 16.8 g
Sugar: 3 g
Sodium: 753 mg

Fiber: 2.9 g

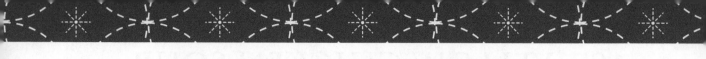

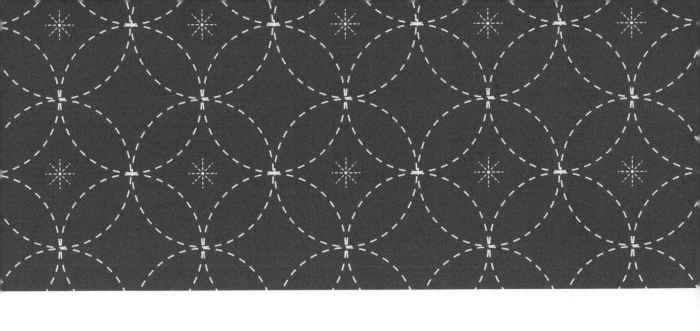

CHAPTER 13
DESSERTS

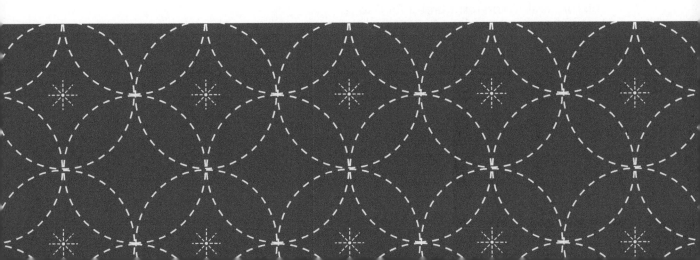

188. CHOCOLATE AVOCADO ICE CREAM

INGREDIENTS

- Large organic avocados, pitted – 2
- Erythritol, powdered – ½ cup
- Cocoa powder, organic and unsweetened – ½ cup
- Drops of liquid stevia – 25
- Vanilla extract, unsweetened – 2 teaspoons
- Coconut milk, full-fat and unsweetened – 1 cup
- Heavy whipping cream, full-fat – ½ cup
- Squares of chocolate, unsweetened and chopped – 6

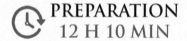 **PREPARATION**
12 H 10 MIN

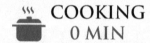 **COOKING**
0 MIN

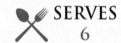 **SERVES**
6

DIRECTIONS

1. Scoop out the flesh from each avocado, place it in a bowl and add vanilla, milk, and cream and blend using an immersion blender until smooth and creamy.
2. Add remaining ingredients except for chocolate and mix until well combined and smooth.
3. Fold in chopped chocolate and let the mixture chill in the refrigerator for 8 to 12 hours or until cooled.
4. When ready to serve, let ice cream stand for 30 minutes at room temperature, then process it using an ice cream machine as per manufacturer instruction.
5. Serve immediately.

Nutritions:

Calories: 216.7 kcal
Fat: 19.4 g
Protein: 3.8 g

Net Carbs: 3.7 g
Fiber: 7.4 g

189. MOCHA MOUSSE

INGREDIENTS

For the Cream Cheese:
- Cream cheese, softened and full-fat – 8 ounces
- Sour cream, full-fat – 3 tablespoons
- Butter, softened – 2 tablespoons
- Vanilla extract, unsweetened – 1 ½ teaspoons
- Erythritol – 1/3 cup
- Cocoa powder, unsweetened – ¼ cup
- Instant coffee powder – 3 teaspoons

For the Whipped Cream:
- Heavy whipping cream, full-fat – 2/3 cup
- Erythritol – 1 ½ teaspoon
- Vanilla extract, unsweetened – ½ teaspoon

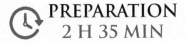 **PREPARATION** 2 H 35 MIN

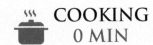 **COOKING** 0 MIN

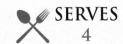 **SERVES** 4

DIRECTIONS

1. Prepare cream cheese mixture: For this, place cream cheese in a bowl, add sour cream and butter then beat until smooth.
2. Now add erythritol, cocoa powder, coffee, and vanilla and blend until incorporated, set aside until required.
3. Prepare whipping cream: For this, place whipping cream in a bowl and beat until soft peaks form.
4. Beat in vanilla and erythritol until stiff peaks form, then add 1/3 of the mixture into cream cheese mixture and fold until just mixed.
5. Then add the remaining whipping cream mixture and fold until evenly incorporated.
6. Spoon the mousse into a freezer-proof bowl and place in the refrigerator for 2 ½ hours until set.
7. Serve straight away.

Nutritions:

Calories: 421.7 kcal
Fat: 42 g
Protein: 6 g

Net Carbs: 6.5 g
Fiber: 2 g

190. PUMPKIN PIE PUDDING

INGREDIENTS

- Eggs – 2
- Heavy whipping cream, divided – 1 cup
- Erythritol sweetener – 3/4 cup
- Pumpkin puree – 15 ounces
- Pumpkin pie spice – 1 teaspoon
- Vanilla extract, unsweetened – 1 teaspoon
- Water – 1 ½ cup

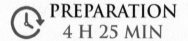 **PREPARATION**
4 H 25 MIN

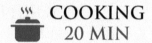 **COOKING**
20 MIN

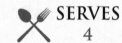 **SERVES**
4

DIRECTIONS

1. Crack eggs in a bowl, add ½ cup cream, sweetener, pumpkin puree, pumpkin pie spice, and vanilla and whisk until blended.
2. Take a 6 by 3-inch baking pan, grease it well with avocado oil, then pour in egg mixture, smooth the top and cover with aluminum foil.
3. Switch on the instant pot, pour in water, insert a trivet stand and place baking pan on it.
4. Shut the instant pot with its lid in the sealed position, then press the 'manual' button, press '+/-' to set the cooking time to 20 minutes and cook at a high-pressure setting; when the pressure builds in the pot, the cooking timer will start.
5. When the instant pot buzzes, press the 'keep warm' button, release pressure naturally for 10 minutes, then do a quick pressure release and open the lid.
6. Take out the baking pan, uncover it, let cool for 15 minutes at room temperature, then transfer the pan into the refrigerator for 4 hours or until cooled.
7. Top pie with remaining cream, then cut it into slices and serve.

Nutritions:

Calories: 184 kcal
Fat: 16 g
Protein: 3 g

Net Carbs: 5 g
Fiber: 2 g

191. AVOCADO & CHOCOLATE PUDDING

INGREDIENTS

- Cream cheese (2 oz.)
- Ripe medium avocado (1)
- Natural sweetener – swerve (1 tsp.)
- Vanilla extract (.25 tsp.)
- Unsweetened cocoa powder (4 tbsp.)
- Pink salt (1 pinch)

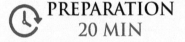 **PREPARATION**
20 MIN

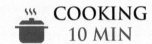 **COOKING**
10 MIN

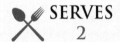 **SERVES**
2

DIRECTIONS

1. Combine the cream cheese with the avocado, sweetener, vanilla, cocoa powder, and salt into the blender or processor.
2. Pulse until creamy smooth.
3. Measure into fancy dessert dishes and chill for at least ½ hour.

Nutritions:

Calories: 281 kcal
Net Carbohydrates: 2 g
Protein: 8 g

Fat Content: 27 g

192. CHEESECAKE PUDDING

INGREDIENTS

- Cream cheese or Neufchatel cheese (1 block)
- Heavy whipping cream (.5 cup)
- Lemon juice (1 tsp.)
- Sour cream (.5 cup)
- Liquid stevia (20 drops)
- Vanilla extract (1 tsp.)

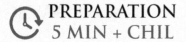 **PREPARATION** 5 MIN + CHIL   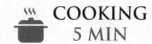 **COOKING** 5 MIN   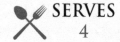 **SERVES** 4

DIRECTIONS

1. Leave the cream cheese on the counter to soften for a few minutes before using.
2. Whip the sour cream and whipping cream together with the mixer until soft peaks form. Combine with the rest of the ingredients and whip until fluffy.
3. Portion into four dishes to chill. Place a layer of the wrap over the dish and store in the fridge.
4. When ready to eat, garnish with some berries if you like.
5. Note: If you add berries, be sure to add the carbs.

Nutritions:

Calories: 356 kcal
Net Carbohydrates: 5 g
Protein: 5 g

Fat Content: 36 g

193. CARROT ALMOND CAKE

INGREDIENTS

- Eggs (3)
- Apple pie spice (1.5 tsp.)
- Almond flour (1 cup)
- Swerve (.66 cup)
- Baking powder (1 tsp.)
- Coconut oil (.25 cup)
- Shredded carrots (1 cup)
- Heavy whipping cream (.5 cup)
- Chopped walnuts (.5 cup)

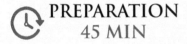 **PREPARATION** 45 MIN

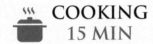 **COOKING** 15 MIN

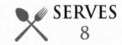 **SERVES** 8

DIRECTIONS

1. Grease cake pan. Combine all of the ingredients with the mixer until well mixed. Pour the mix into the pan and cover with a layer of foil.
2. Pour two cups of water into the Instant Pot bowl along with the steamer rack.
3. Arrange the pan on the trivet and set the pot using the cake button (40 min.).
4. Natural-release the pressure for ten minutes. Then, quick-release the rest of the built-up steam pressure.
5. Cool then start frosting or serve it plain.

Nutritions:

Calories: 268 kcal Protein: 6 g
Net Carbohydrates: 4 g
Fat Content: 25 g

194. CHOCOLATE LAVA CAKE

INGREDIENTS

- Unsweetened cocoa powder (.5 cup)
- Melted butter (.25 cup)
- Eggs (4)
- Sugar-free chocolate sauce (.25 cup)
- Sea salt (.5 tsp.)
- Ground cinnamon (.5 tsp.)
- Pure vanilla extract (1 tsp.)
- Stevia (.25 cup)
- Also Needed: Ice cube tray & 4 ramekins

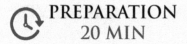 **PREPARATION**
20 MIN

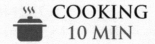 **COOKING**
10 MIN

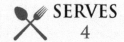 **SERVES**
4

DIRECTIONS

1. Pour one tablespoon of the chocolate sauce into four of the tray slots and freeze.
2. Warm up the oven to 350° Fahrenheit. Lightly grease the ramekins with butter or a spritz of oil.
3. Mix the salt, cinnamon, cocoa powder, and stevia until combined. Whisk in the eggs – one at a time. Stir in the melted vanilla extract and butter.
4. Fill each of the ramekins halfway and add one of the frozen chocolates. Cover the rest of the container with the cake batter.
5. Bake for 13-14 minutes. When they're set, place them on a wire rack to cool for about five minutes. Remove and put on a serving dish.
6. Enjoy by slicing its molten center.

Nutritions:

Calories: 189 kcal
Net Carbohydrates: 3 g
Protein: 8 g

Fat Content: 17 g

195. GLAZED POUND CAKE

INGREDIENTS

- Salt (.5 tsp.)
- Almond flour (2.5 cups)
- Softened - unsalted butter (.5 cup)
- Erythritol (1.5 cups)
- Unchilled eggs (8)
- Lemon extract (.5 tsp.)
- Vanilla extract (1.5 tsp.)
- Cream cheese (8 oz.)
- Baking powder (1.5 tsp.)
- The Glaze:
- Powdered erythritol (.25 cup)
- Heavy whipping cream (3 tbsp.)

- Vanilla extract (.5 tsp.)

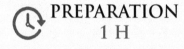 **PREPARATION**
1 H

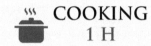 **COOKING**
1 H

 **SERVES**
16

DIRECTIONS

1. Warm the oven to 350° Fahrenheit.
2. Whisk together baking powder, almond flour, and salt
3. Cream the erythritol, butter, and softened cream cheese chunks. Mix until smooth in a large mixing container.
4. Whisk and add the eggs with the lemon and vanilla extract. Blend with the rest of the ingredients using a hand mixer until smooth.
5. Dump the batter into a loaf pan. Bake for one to two hours.
6. Prepare a glaze. Mix in the vanilla extract, powdered erythritol, and heavy whipping cream until smooth.
7. You must let the cake cool completely before adding the glaze.

Nutritions:

Calories: 254 kcal
Net Carbohydrates: 2.5 g
Protein: 7.9 g

Fat Content: 23.4 g

196. LEMON CAKE

INGREDIENTS

- Coconut flour (.5 cup)
- Baking powder (2 tsp.)
- Almond flour (1.5 cups)
- Swerve (or) Pyure A-P (3 tbsp.)
- Optional: Xanthan gum (.5 tsp.)
- Whipping cream (.5 cup)
- Melted butter (.5 cup)
- Zest & juice (2 lemons)
- Eggs (2)

Ingredients for the Topping:
- Pyure all-purpose/Swerve (3 tbsp.)
- Lemon juice (2 tbsp.)
- Boiling water (.5 cup)
- Melted butter (2 tbsp.)
- Suggested: 2-4-quart slow cooker

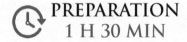 **PREPARATION**
1 H 30 MIN

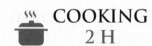 **COOKING**
2 H

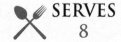 **SERVES**
8

DIRECTIONS

1. For the Cake: Mix the dry ingredients in a container. Whisk the egg with the lemon juice and zest, butter, and whipping cream. Whisk all of the ingredients and scoop out the dough into the prepared slow cooker.
2. For the Topping: Mix all of the topping ingredients in a container and empty over the batter in the cooker.
3. Place the lid on the cooker for two to three hours on the high setting.
4. Serve warm with some fresh fruit or whipped cream.

Nutritions:

Calories: 350 kcal *Fat Content: 33 g*
Net Carbohydrates: 5.2 g
Protein: 7.6 g

197. SPICE CAKES

INGREDIENTS

- Salted butter (.5 cup)
- Erythritol (.75 cup)
- Eggs (4 - divided)
- Vanilla extract (1 tsp.)
- Ground cloves (.25 tsp.)
- Baking powder (2 tsp.)
- Allspice (.5 tsp.)
- Nutmeg (.5 tsp.
- Almond flour (2 cups)
- Cinnamon (.5 tsp.)
- Ginger (.5 tsp.)
- Water (5 tbsp.)

- Also Needed: Cupcake tray

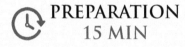 **PREPARATION**
15 MIN

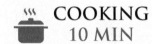 **COOKING**
10 MIN

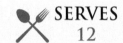 **SERVES**
12

DIRECTIONS

1. Warm the oven temperature to 350° Fahrenheit. Prepare the baking tray with liners (12).
2. Mix the butter and erythritol with a hand mixer. Once it's smooth, combine with two eggs and the vanilla. Add the rest of the eggs and mix well.
3. Grind the clove to a fine powder and add with the rest of the spices. Whisk into the mixture. Stir in the baking powder and almond flour. Blend in the water. When the batter is smooth, add to the prepared tin.
4. Bake for 15 minutes. Enjoy any time.

Nutritions:

Calories: 277 kcal
Net Carbohydrates: 3 g
Protein: 6 g

Fat Content: 27 g

198. VANILLA - SOUR CREAM CUPCAKES

INGREDIENTS

- Butter (4 tbsp.)
- Swerve or your favorite sweetener (1.5 cups)
- Salt (.25 tsp.)
- Eggs (4)
- Sour cream (.25 cup)
- Vanilla (1 tsp.)
- Almond flour (1 cup)
- Baking powder (1 tsp.)
- Coconut flour (.25 cup)

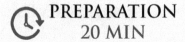 **PREPARATION**
20 MIN

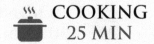 **COOKING**
25 MIN

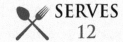 **SERVES**
12

DIRECTIONS

1. Warm the oven at 350° Fahrenheit.
2. Prepare the butter and sweetener until creamy and fluffy using the mixer.
3. Blend in the vanilla and sour cream. Mix well.
4. One at a time, fold in the eggs.
5. Sift and blend in both types of flour, salt, and baking powder.
6. Divide the batter between the cups.
7. Bake for 20 to 25 minutes. Times may vary according to your oven hotness.
8. Cool completely and place in the fridge for fresher results.

Nutritions:

Calories: 128 kcal   Protein: 4 g
Net Carbohydrates: 2 g
Fat Content: 11 g

199. BROWNED BUTTER CHOCOLATE CHIP BLONDIES

INGREDIENTS

- Butter (.5 cup)
- Almond flour (2 cups)
- Swerve sweetener (.25 cup)
- Baking powder (1 tsp.)
- Salt (.5 tsp.)
- Sukrin Gold (.25 cup) or more swerve + molasses (2 tsp.)
- Large egg (1)
- Sugar-free chocolate chips (.33 cup)
- Vanilla extract (.5 tsp.)
- Also Needed: 9x9-inch baking pan

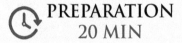 **PREPARATION** 20 MIN   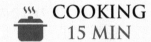 **COOKING** 15 MIN   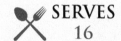 **SERVES** 16

DIRECTIONS

1. Set the oven temperature at 325° Fahrenheit. Lightly grease the pan.
2. Toss the butter into the pan using the medium temperature setting. Cook until the butter is melted and becomes a deep amber (4-5 min.).
3. Remove the pan from the burner to cool.
4. Whisk the almond flour with the salt, baking powder, and sweeteners.
5. Whisk the egg and add it to the mixture with the browned butter and vanilla extract until thoroughly combined. Fold in the chocolate chips.
6. Press the dough evenly into the prepared pan.
7. Set a timer to bake for 15-20 minutes or until just set and golden brown.
8. Let the blondies cool in the pan. Slice into squares and serve as desired.

Nutritions:

Calories: 161 kcal
Net Carbohydrates: 3 g
Protein: 3.8 g

Fat Content: 14.4 g

200. CHOCOLATE CHIP COOKIES

INGREDIENTS

- Eggs (2 large)
- Melted butter (1 stick - .5 cup)
- Pure vanilla extract - alcohol-free (2 tsp.)
- Heavy cream (2 tbsp.)
- Almond flour (2.75 cups)
- Kosher salt (.25 tsp.)
- Swerve (.5 cup or to taste)
- Dark chocolate chips - ex. Lily's (.75 cup)
- Cooking spray - as needed

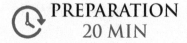 **PREPARATION** 20 MIN
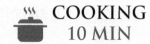 **COOKING** 10 MIN
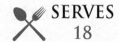 **SERVES** 18

DIRECTIONS

1. Set the oven temperature at 350° Fahrenheit. Prepare the pan.
2. Whisk the egg with the heavy cream, butter, vanilla, almond flour, salt, and swerve.
3. Fold the chocolate chips into the batter.
4. Form the mixture into one-inch balls. Flatten the balls with the glass or your hands that's been lightly greased with cooking spray.
5. Arrange the cookies about three inches apart on the cookie sheets.
6. Bake until the cookies are golden, about 17-19 minutes.

Nutritions:

Calories: 96 kcal
Net Carbohydrates: 1 g
Protein: 2 g

Fat Content: 9 g

201. KEY LIME BARS

INGREDIENTS

The Crust:
- Almond flour (1.25 cups)
- Swerve Sweetener (.33 cup)
- Salt (.25 tsp.)
- Melted butter (.25 cup)

The Filling:
- Unchilled cream cheese (3 oz. - softened)
- Lime zest (2 tsp.)
- Sugar-free condensed milk (1 cup)
- Egg yolks (4)
- Key lime juice (6 tbsp.)
- Also Suggested: 8x8-inch baking pan

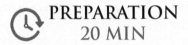 **PREPARATION** 20 MIN

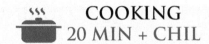 **COOKING** 20 MIN + CHIL

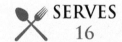 **SERVES** 16

DIRECTIONS

The Crust:
1. Warm the oven to 325° Fahrenheit.
2. Whisk the almond flour with the salt and sweetener.
3. Melt the butter and add to the mixture to make the batter.
4. Pour the batter into the pan. Press firmly into the bottom.
5. Bake until just golden brown around the edges (for 12-15 min.).
6. Transfer to the countertop to cool.

The Key Lime:
7. Beat the cream cheese and lime zest until creamy smooth.
8. Whisk and fold in the egg yolks until well mixed.
9. Slowly pour in the juice from the lime and condensed milk. Stir until the filling is creamy smooth.
10. Add the filling into the crust. Bake it for 15-20 minutes.
11. Remove and cool. Store in the fridge for one hour to set.
12. Top with lightly sweetened whipped cream and lime slices if desired.

Nutritions:

Calories: 188 kcal
Net Carbohydrates: 2.4 g
Protein: 3.4 g

Fat Content: 17.5 g

202. RASPBERRY FUDGE

INGREDIENTS

- Cream cheese (16 oz.)
- Butter (1 cup)
- White sugar substitute (.25 cup)
- Unsweetened cocoa powder (6 tbsp.)
- Heavy cream (2 tbsp.)
- Vanilla extract (2 tsp.)
- Raspberry extract (1 tsp.)
- Chopped walnuts (.33 cup)

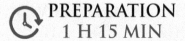 **PREPARATION**
1 H 15 MIN

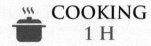 **COOKING**
1 H

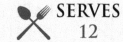 **SERVES**
12

DIRECTIONS

1. Mix the cream cheese and butter in the mixing bowl with the mixer.
2. When smooth, mix with the rest of the ingredients until well incorporated.
3. Microwave using the high setting for 30 seconds. Blend with the mixer again until smooth.
4. Empty into the prepared pan (1-inch layer). Cover and chill for two hours in the fridge.
5. Slice into 12 portions.
6. Serve and enjoy or store in the fridge for a delicious treat later.

Nutritions:

Calories: 242 kcal   Fat Content: 25.3 g
Net Carbohydrates: 4.4 g
Protein: 2.6 g

203. SUNFLOWER SEED SURPRISE COOKIES

INGREDIENTS

- Egg (50 g/1 large egg)
- Sugar-free sunflower seed butter (100 g/.75 cup)
- Coconut oil (16 g/1 rounded tbsp.)
- Optional: Truvia (12 g/1 tbsp.)
- Vanilla extract (2 g/.5 tsp.)
- Salt - Baking powder & soda (1 g/1 pinch each)

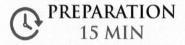 **PREPARATION** 15 MIN
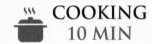 **COOKING** 10 MIN
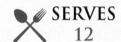 **SERVES** 12

DIRECTIONS

1. Warm the oven temperature setting to 350° Fahrenheit. Set the rack in the upper portion of the oven.
2. Prepare a cookie tray using a layer of parchment baking paper.
3. Mix all of the ingredients in a large container.
4. Roll and flatten the mixture into 12 balls about the width of a quarter.
5. Bake the cookies for seven to nine minutes until they're firm in the center.
6. Cool the cookies for a couple of hours.

Nutritions:

Calories: 69 kcal
Net Carbohydrates: 0.64 g
Protein: 2.3 g

Fat Content: 6.3 g

204. KETO PIE CRUST

INGREDIENTS

- Salt (.25 tsp.)
- Butter - melted (.25 cup)

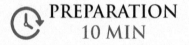 **PREPARATION**
10 MIN

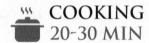 **COOKING**
20-30 MIN

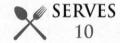 **SERVES**
10

DIRECTIONS

1. Whisk the salt, sweetener, and flour in a mixing container. Fold in the melted butter to form coarse crumbs.
2. Dump it into a pie plate and press it firmly to the sides and bottom. Prick it using a toothpick or fork.
3. For unfilled Crust: Bake 325° Fahrenheit for about 20 minutes.
4. For filled Crust: Pre-bake it for 10-12 minutes before adding the ingredients. Cover the edges to avoid over-browning.

Nutritions:

Calories: 187 kcal
Net Carbohydrates: 1.8 g
Fat Content: 12.7 g

Protein: 3.7 g

205. DELICIOUS CHEESECAKE

INGREDIENTS

- Eggs (2)
- Vanilla extract (2 tsp.)
- Sour cream (1.5 cups)
- Splenda granules/another keto-friendly sweetener (.5 cup)
- Unchilled cream cheese (16 oz.)
- Melted butter (2 tbsp.)
- Also Needed: 12 ramekins or 10-inch springform pan

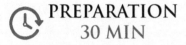 **PREPARATION** 30 MIN 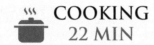 **COOKING** 22 MIN 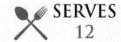 **SERVES** 12

DIRECTIONS

1. Warm the oven temperature at 350° Fahrenheit.
2. Whisk the eggs, vanilla, sour cream, and Splenda in a large mixing container. Work in the cream cheese and butter.
3. Spoon and combine about ½ cup of the mixture into another bowl and add the raspberry flavoring.
4. Spoon the rest of the mix into the chosen container.
5. Scoop a spoon of the raspberry batter over the top. Swirl it through the plain mixture.
6. Prepare a crust from ¼ cup of Splenda, ¼ cup of butter, and 1 ½ cup ground almonds. Mix it like a graham cracker crust and add it to the ramekins/pan.
7. Arrange the ramekins in a water bath (a shallow pan with water) in the oven below the ramekins/pan.
8. Bake for 20-25 minutes for ramekins or 35-40 minutes in a springform pan. The cake will firm up when refrigerated.
9. Top it off using raspberries and whipped cream - but add the carbs. Freeze if desired.

Note: The nutritional calculations do not include crust.

Nutritions:

Calories: 231.8 kcal
Net Carbohydrates: 3.4 g
Protein: 4.9 g

Fat Content: 22.3 g

206. COCOA BROWNIES

INGREDIENTS

- ½ c salted butter, melted
- 1 c Granular Swerve Sweetener
- 2 Large Eggs
- 2 t vanilla extract
- squares unsweetened baking chocolate, melted
- 2 T coconut flour
- 2 T cocoa powder
- ½ T baking powder
- ½ t salt
- ½ c walnuts, chopped (optional)

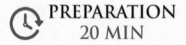 **PREPARATION**
20 MIN

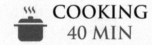 **COOKING**
40 MIN

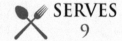 **SERVES**
9

DIRECTIONS

1. Preheat oven to 350 degrees.
2. Spray square baking pan with cooking spray or grease pan well with butter.
3. In a large mixing bowl, use an electric mixer or whisk and mix together butter and sweetener.
4. Add the eggs and vanilla extract to the bowl and mix with an electric mixer for 1 minute until smooth.
5. Add melted chocolate and stir with a wooden spoon or spatula until the chocolate is incorporated into the butter mixture.
6. In a separate bowl, mix the dry ingredients (remaining ingredients besides walnuts) until combined.
7. Add dry ingredients into the bowl with the wet ingredients and stir with a wooden spoon until combined.
8. Add walnuts if desired.
9. Pour batter into prepared pan. Spread to cover the entire bottom of the pan and into corners.
10. Place in the center rack of the oven and bake for 30 minutes.
11. After the brownies are baked, take them out and leave them in the pan to cool.
12. When cool, cut them into 9 servings, and they are ready to eat.

These have to be a once-in-a-while treat because they are sweet, and if you're like me, that sugar will continue to call your name. These are so good you will have to work to eat only one serving.

Nutritions:

Calories: 201 kcal   Fat: 19 g
Carbohydrates: 5 g
Protein: 3 g

207. KETO BROWN BUTTER PRALINES

INGREDIENTS

- 2 Sticks Salted butter
- 2/3 c heavy cream
- 2/3 c monk fruit sweetener
- ½ t xanthan gum
- 2 c pecans, chopped
- Sea salt

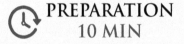 **PREPARATION**
10 MIN

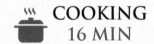 **COOKING**
16 MIN

 **SERVES**
10

DIRECTIONS

1. Line a cookie sheet with parchment paper or use a silicone baking mat.
2. Prepare a cookie sheet with parchment paper or a silicone baking mat.
3. In a medium-size, medium weight saucepan, brown the butter until it smells nutty. Don't burn the butter. This will take about 5 minutes.
4. Stir in heavy cream, xanthan gum, and sweetener.
5. Take the pan off the heat and stir in the nuts.
6. Place pan in the refrigerator for an hour.
7. Stir the mixture occasionally while it is getting colder.
8. After an hour, scoop the mixture onto the cookie sheets and shape it into cookies.
9. Sprinkle with sea salt.
10. Refrigerate on the cookie sheet until the pralines are hard.
11. After the cookies are hard, transfer them to an airtight container in the refrigerator.

This is a special treat. A low carb praline with the fat from the butter and cream. It is a nice dessert to have on a special occasion that you can work into your day without totally messing up your macros. The monk fruit sweetener is a 1:1 measure, so the texture is not altered by not using sugar. Give them a try and you will not be disappointed.

Nutritions:

Calories: 338 kcal
Carbohydrates: 1 g
Protein: 2 g

Fat: 36 g

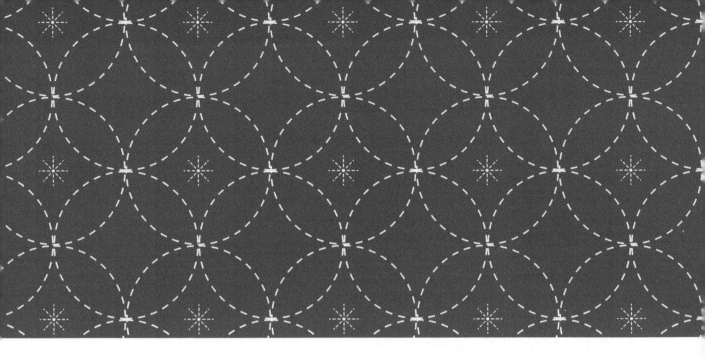

CONCLUSION

Your dedication to improve your health and lose weight is phenomenal since you have been able to reach the end of this book. It is not an easy process to lose weight if you will be able to maintain the guidelines you have learned in this book and stay motivated; your life will change in ways that you cannot imagine. You are on the right track to achieve both mental and physical health. Even though adjusting to eating a healthy diet after being accustomed to eating a lot of convenience foods is a challenge, you will feel the difference in energy levels that you will experience. You will look good and be safe from many of the common nutrition-related diseases and conditions and on top of all of that; your quality of life will improve greatly.

We are all different; thus, you should take time to really understand what a weight loss program involves and try out the program gradually. If you nose dive into a weight loss program is not advisable since it may not be for you. No regiment works perfectly for everyone; thus, you should select a plan and modify it in a way that suits you. There are many weight loss programs with mind-blowing results, but they may be too hard to follow or just unsafe to practice.

The intensity, duration and rest period are factors that must be taken into account. It best works when it is a constant in your daily activity and as it is not a permanent change of your physical and psychological condition.

In order to get the maximum weight loss experience, you should listen to your body. This does not mean that you should eat any time you feel hungry, it means that you should listen to how it responds to your diet and fasting regiment because the body system determines the time for you to eat, time for you to exercise and even how many calories you take in. Thus, you will be in full control of your weight loss once you are in control of your diet and fasting program.

You should know that even though the ketogenic diet is about carbohydrate restriction, do not excessively restrict them you should make sure you eat enough. If you restrict calories too much you will be moody and it can even stop your fat loss process. You should also vary your food choices so that you make sure that you are getting the nutrients you need so as to maintain your health.

In fact, getting all the nutrients that you require from a ketogenic diet is possible. Unfortunately for some, this is not possible. If you do not feel okay, you should go and see a doctor so as to determine if you have any nutritional deficiencies. He/she will able to recommend supplements for you from that information.

For health reasons, weight loss should be a slow process. Losing 2 pounds a day is okay, but anything more than that is a lot. Engage in your day-to-day operations while fasting as this is a time-flying route. Good luck on your keto diet journey!

INDEX OF RECIPES

CPSIA information can be obtained
at www.ICGtesting.com
Printed in the USA
BVHW011336270622
640728BV00008B/291